Advance Praise for *Reflecting on the Inevitable*

"Is it possible to comprehend one's own death? Might the attempt to do so be critical for the engagement with one's own life? *Reflecting on the Inevitable* takes the reader on a journey into the midst of the questions that emerge here, drawing together a range of philosophical and psychological considerations within an intriguing and accessible narrative that will be of value, not only to students and researchers in many different fields, but also to anyone who has begun to reflect on the fact of their own inevitable demise."

—**Jeff Malpas, PhD, FAHA,** Emeritus Distinguished Professor,
University of Tasmania, Tasmania, Australia

"This is a rich and fascinating study of the prospect of personal death. The book is unusual in that it combines insights from various different disciplines and schools of thought. Adams' discussions are thought-provoking and more entertaining than the subject matter might suggest."

—**Jens Johansson, PhD,** Professor of Philosophy,
Uppsala University, Uppsala, Sweden

"*Reflecting on the Inevitable* provides an accessible and interdisciplinary guide to the philosophy and psychology of death. Adams' focus on personal mortality makes this book an especially welcome contribution to the literature. It will be of interest to anyone with a serious interest in the personal dimension of mortality as well as the general issue of how we may think our way through this extremely elusive realm of human experience."

—**Paul Fairfield, PhD,** Professor of Philosophy,
Queen's University, Kingston, Ontario, Canada

"Adams' highly original, sensitive, attention to the struggle we each have with our own death resulted in a finely tuned, delicately argued book. It uses the literary aid of four fictional characters, whose presence in the book makes its ideas both accessible and engaging."

—**Havi Carel, PhD,** Professor of Philosophy, University of Bristol, Bristol, England, United Kingdom

Reflecting on the Inevitable

Mortality at the Crossroads of Psychology, Philosophy, and Health

PETER J. ADAMS, PhD

Professor, School of Population Health
University of Auckland
Auckland, New Zealand

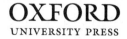

OXFORD
UNIVERSITY PRESS

OXFORD
UNIVERSITY PRESS

Oxford University Press is a department of the University of Oxford. It furthers the University's objective of excellence in research, scholarship, and education by publishing worldwide. Oxford is a registered trade mark of Oxford University Press in the UK and certain other countries.

Published in the United States of America by Oxford University Press
198 Madison Avenue, New York, NY 10016, United States of America.

© Oxford University Press 2020

Library of Congress Cataloging-in-Publication Data
Names: Adams, Peter J., 1956– author.
Title: Reflecting on the inevitable : mortality at the crossroads of psychology, philosophy, and health / Peter J. Adams.
Description: New York, NY : Oxford University Press, 2020. |
Includes bibliographical references and index.
Identifiers: LCCN 2019044709 (print) | LCCN 2019044710 (ebook) |
ISBN 9780190945008 (paperback) | ISBN 9780190945022 (epub) |
ISBN 9780190945039 (electronic)
Subjects: MESH: Attitude to Death
Classification: LCC BF789.D4 (print) | LCC BF789.D4 (ebook) |
NLM BF 789.D4 | DDC 155.9/37—dc23
LC record available at https://lccn.loc.gov/2019044709
LC ebook record available at https://lccn.loc.gov/2019044710

1 3 5 7 9 8 6 4 2

Printed by Marquis, Canada

Contents

Preface   vii
Acknowledgments   ix
Introduction   xi

1. Other People Die   1

2. My-Death   20

3. Limits of Intelligibility   34

4. Aversion and Evasion   48

5. A Constant Companion   67

6. Essential Structures   85

7. Passionate Suffusion   103

8. Point-of-Transition   124

9. Self-Generative Process   145

10. Dialogue   162

11. What's to Gain?   178

12. Applications   197

Conclusion   216

Bibliography   221
Index   235

Preface

Whenever I try to think about my own death I end up muddled and confused. Given the importance of the topic, this is disappointing, and it puts me off thinking about death any further.

Despite this disappointment, I do sometimes manage to pursue such thoughts through to a level that seems to make some sort of sense or, at least, gives me some way of talking about it. But then, just when I seem to be making progress, I push things a bit further and the framework of ideas begins to crumble. Then I take one step further and the whole edifice collapses. What I'm thinking becomes nonsensical, and I'm left with no clues as to how to move on. In my frustration I back away. I resolve to avoid thinking about it again or, at least, to avoid it until I've managed to forget what happened previously.

So, let's take a closer look at the usual sequence. I typically start by imagining what it would be like to be in the shoes of someone I know who had just died. I then project my experience into what I imagine would be the experience of that person as they approached their death. Maybe it would be my consciousness that expires like a light that has permanently been switched off. Maybe it would be my body lying motionless in the coffin. Maybe it would be my soul that is absorbed into a zone of endless tranquility.

I next take this idea of me as the dead person and visualize myself approaching a border zone, a point of transition, a place where the world of everyday life is divided from some form of afterlife: perhaps to a place beyond—a place up there, under here, or in another dimension—perhaps to a place that souls inhabit such as paradise or heaven, or perhaps even a place of open possibilities, a realm of indeterminacy where individual identity is subsumed into a collective identity.

Coupled with this idea of transition to an afterlife is the idea of my death entailing some form of absence. As I continue to project my existence—or nonexistence—onto this other person, I imagine other people in my life reacting to my departure. I conjure up images of loved ones with shocked expressions as they are told about my death, I visualize their forlorn looks as they watch my coffin descending into the grave, and I picture their reactions to constantly interacting with the spaces I now no longer occupy. I know these reactions well because it's what I've experienced when others close to me have died.

But hold on: thinking about my mortality in terms of what happens to others when they die does not fully capture what happens when I think about my own death. When I, the individual doing my experiencing, die, my consciousness, as normally understood, draws to a close. I am no longer present to observe what is going on. I cease to be part of the world.

The trouble is that my own death and the deaths of other people are not equivalent. When other people die I can watch it happen and interpret their death as an absence of what had previously existed. When it comes to my own death, I don't have the vantage point from which to interpret it as an absence. My own death brings with it the finality of my consciousness, and, as a consequence, it places at risk the whole notion of a continuing world. What is at stake with the end of my consciousness is the total annihilation of everything. Identifying an absence only makes sense when it is contrasted with some form of continuity. My death threatens this continuity and thereby disrupts any attempt to use what I understand about the death of others to make sense of my own death.

But hold on again: How can I be sure this is what it's like? Even the notion of world-minus-my-consciousness assumes that something persists in which my absence is able to register. Annihilation only makes sense against some form of backdrop, even if it is a persisting blackness or void. Something still needs to be there for finality and annihilation to be enacted.

So, how on earth can I begin to think and speak about the possibility of my own death when, whatever concepts I use, they somehow still assume some form of continuation?

It is at this point that everything collapses. My thoughts are swirling into a self-consuming vortex where my ideas about death have become disoriented and nonsensical. I lack any secure foundation on which to build, and I find myself unpleasantly overwhelmed by this spinning maelstrom. I resolve not to allow myself to think in this direction again. But is it a waste of time?

Acknowledgments

Books are seldom written in isolation from surrounding influences and supports, so, before continuing, I want to acknowledge a few people whose generosity made this work possible. First, I want to thank my friend and colleague John Raeburn for our ongoing conversations, for his feedback on draft chapters, and for his willingness to read and comment on the first complete draft. Next, I am grateful to my New Zealand Society of Authors colleague, Bernard Brown, for his kind offer to read a draft and provide feedback.

I am grateful for the many supportive conversations I had with colleagues leading up to writing the book, particularly those with Monique Jonas, Rachel Simon-Kumar, and Yvonne Bray. I am also grateful for the stimulating conversations I had with death scholars in England, especially the lively conversations with Douglas Davies at Durham University and with Julie Rugg and Ruth Penfold-Mounce at the University of York. Thanks also for the patient support of the editors at Oxford University Press, particularly Marta Moldvai and Tiffany Lu.

In terms of broader influences, the key people I would like to acknowledge are my philosophy teachers in the 1970s, particularly Clive Pearson and Bernard Pflaum, both who have sadly passed away. I also wish to acknowledge my employer, the University of Auckland, for granting me six months research and study leave during which I wrote this book.

I am particularly grateful to my wife, Judith, and children, Emily, William, Josie, and Steph, for putting up with my physical and mental absences when engrossed with developing the book. Also, a special thank you to my mother, Nelly, for providing a writing space in the "old house" and the many conversations we had over lunch.

Introduction

An interest in personal mortality may appear curious. There are plenty of other aspects of death that warrant attention. Current research and scholarship in death studies is rapidly expanding and includes a wide array of topics, such as the process of dying, responses to grief and bereavement, caring for the dying, cultural practices surrounding death, our ongoing fear of death, conceptual understandings of death, and how death beliefs relate to religious and philosophical perspectives.[1] So why choose personal mortality, the most elusive and difficult topic of them all?

My own mortality, or "my-death" as it will be called from now on, has accompanied me throughout life.[2] Every now and then my-death hints at its presence and I am forced to reflect on its potency. During such reflections I am daunted by the sheer impenetrability of what to make of it. These moments happen often enough to generate a vague sense that my-death is always there. Indeed, this is the central argument of the book. I will present the case that, from the moment of our birth, whether we like it or not, we enter into an ongoing relationship with my-death. Sometimes the relationship is conscious and visible, at other times it fades into the background; either way, my-death strides alongside us in the form of a continuous presence, a constant companion. The tricky bit is finding some way of thinking and talking about this relationship.

The elusive nature of my-death makes it difficult to separate it out as a discrete focus from other aspects of death. For example, the way loved ones die is likely to influence how we think about our own mortality. Nonetheless, for the purposes of this book, I intend to peel my-death away from other aspects of death so we can focus specifically on what it means in our lives. I plan to do this by means of two important distinctions: one regarding the difference between my-death and dying and another regarding the difference between my-death and the death of other people, or "other-death."

First, the way we understand "dying," and more specifically my-dying, needs to be thought of differently from the way we understand "death" and my-death. Dying occurs as an event in life; it is the process of arriving at death and as such refers to all the pain and adjustment that the dying person and surrounding loved ones experience during those final days and hours. Death, on the other hand, is not confined to that point at which each of us dies. Admittedly, our relationship to death is more strongly highlighted at this point, but it extends beyond dying. Death is a possibility throughout life, and, accordingly, its presence permeates day-to-day life on an ongoing basis.[3] This can be seen with someone who has reached a point where death no longer concerns them; death is peacefully welcomed and accepted, but, at the same time, this person might perceive the process of dying as something worrying and frightening. As distinct from dying as an event in life, death points toward more fundamental structures and relationships that permeate throughout life.

The second critical distinction concerns the difference between my own death ("my-death") and other people's deaths ("other-death"). The significance of this difference will be revisited multiple times in various parts of the book. When other people die we not only observe how this occurs, but we are also able to observe what happens afterward. We can watch how the absence of the deceased unfolds within the nexus of their family and friendship relationships. When it comes to my-death, we are not able to observe what happens afterward because the conditions for observing, such as consciousness and sensory perception, are no longer available. We might try to think of my-death as resembling other-death by conjuring up images of our absence continuing in a world that carries on, but such images are extensions of how we understand other-death and are not based on what we understand as my-death. In other words, other-death belongs to what is recognizable in life, whereas my-death connects us with something that lies beyond recognition: perhaps to the nothingness of nonexistence or to the annihilation of all consciousness.

The book has been organized into the form of a journey that ventures into unpredictable and volatile territories. The journey starts out in the swamp of conceptual uncertainty which surrounds personal mortality; it then traverses several islands of possibility and finally ends up on a peninsular looking out at my-death as a vital and life-enhancing relationship permeating one's whole being. The journey can be further subdivided into five legs, with each leg shaped by particular problems or particular tasks. The first leg—consisting of Chapters 1 and 2—explores in more detail the difference between other-death and my-death. While much of what we seem to know about my-death is derived from what we observe about the death of others, on closer inspection, the applicability of these observations begin to break down. Chapter 2 then proceeds to explore how far thinking about my-death might go; how far the concept can be pushed before it reaches the bounds of intelligibility.

The second leg—consisting of Chapters 3 and 4—focuses on the incomprehensibility of one's own mortality and the fear that arises from not knowing how to think about it. It begins with claims that my-death marks the cessation of consciousness, the end of everything, and the prospect of total annihilation. It contends that these fall far short of an adequate conceptualization of my-death because they are derived from how we see things behaving within our lives. Their coherence falls apart when trying to apply it outside our lives. The second part, Chapter 4, then explores what we know about our avoidance of my-death and the various ways we evade thinking and talking about it.

The third leg is made up of one pivotal chapter, Chapter 5, in which the central problem skirted around in previous chapters, the unspeakable and incomprehensible character of my-death, is directly confronted. It concludes that, indeed, we have no clear way of thinking and speaking about my-death, and yet we still see it as important and we still seek out ways of maintaining a personal relationship with it. The chapter proposes that we can access a range of convenient conceptual devices which, though their veracity is beyond appraisal, can act as provisional platforms, as "enabling frames," which provide a mechanism for positioning ourselves in a relationship with my-death.

The fourth leg consists of five chapters—Chapters 6 to 10—which explore the merits of four specific enabling frames as examples of what an ongoing and livable relationship to my-death might look like. Each of these frames—essential structures, passionate suffusion, point-of-transition, and self-generative process—are built around a distinct central idea which is then supported by a complex of related beliefs, metaphors, and other communicative devices. The last chapter in this leg, Chapter 10, talks over the relative merits of all four frames and examines their implications for daily living.

The fifth and final leg, Chapters 11 and 12, focuses on the consequences of pursuing an ongoing relationship with my-death. Chapter 11 addresses questions regarding what might be gained by engaging in a relationship with my-death: Does it improve our quality of life? Does it help us clarify fundamental values? Does it help us prepare for our end of life? I will contend that it can achieve all of these. Finally, Chapter 12 explores how ideas from the book might be applied in practical ways to promoting my-death awareness more generally. Certainly, one chapter on practical applications is hardly sufficient, but conceptual work on the nature of my-death required more attention. The most that can be expected in this limited space is an overview of future possibilities that could then be explored in more detail at a later time.

Before venturing further, I want to introduce four characters: Leo, Mandy, Stan, and Brenda. They will be accompanying us on our journey and will actively contribute to each section of the book. As characters, they are not crafted in the way characters are developed in novels or films. They have been assembled because they represent connections to my-death at different ages and because they are each concurrently grappling with significant transitions in their relationships with my-death. In real life it is very unlikely for four people to be simultaneously preoccupied with death and even less likely for them to be talking openly about their dilemmas. Their conversations could be seen as unnecessarily contrived and slavishly aligned to the intentions of each chapter. To circumvent this, I am inviting you to suspend judgment on the likelihood of these interactions and allow them to form a presence so the characters can contribute in a lively way to the main thrust of the book. At times the characters will introduce new ideas; at other times they will disagree with each other, thereby highlighting the complexities of the issues; and, at other times they will connect these issues to common challenges in everyday life. They will, in a sense, be the layers of flesh providing human context to the dry bones of the conceptual skeleton of the book. The following passage introduces each of them along with the environment in which they will be interacting.[4]

Around the corner of the house and into the back yard strode Leo. The bounce in his legs signaled both the abundant energy packed into his nineteen-year-old body and his eagerness to get things done. Behind him, Stan, a man in his early eighties, was puffing as he struggled to keep up with his youthful guide.

"It's back here. I've put it on the table so we can inspect it." Leo pointed at the lawnmower sitting on newspapers he'd laid out across the garden table, "but I don't really know what to do . . . then I remembered you'd served in the military; you must have fixed dozens of machines."

Stan looked forward to his unpredictable interactions with Leo; he loved his energy and constant flow of ideas. But he worried that Leo might hold him in too high regard. He hadn't told him how, when serving in the army, he'd had practically no experience fixing engines . . . still, he might be able to help. He bent forward and, leaning from side to side, he inspected the mower. It was an old machine and had seen better days.

Stan creaked his body awkwardly upright. He coughed, then glanced across at Leo. "It's best to eliminate the easy problems first." He unscrewed the gas cap, looked in, nodded, screwed it shut, then checked the oil. "Well, that's all okay. Now, what about the sparkplug?"

"Ah, okay, but I don't know how to get to it."

"It's easy, but it's best if you have the right tool," stated Stan authoritatively. "I just happen to have a sparkplug wrench in my tool shed, and, if you wait a bit, I'll bring it over."

Leo watched Stan shuffle slowly back along the side of the house heading for his shed next door. He lifted his gaze to watch his mother, Mandy, moving about in the kitchen. He had a sudden thought, "Oh, I forgot." His mother had told him a new boarder would be arriving this afternoon. He sat down on a chair and continued his scrutiny of his mother's movements. "She's tidying everything up . . . she's always so busy . . . I wish we didn't need boarders . . . but I know that without them we'd struggle to survive and I would have to stop going to college." He continued to watch her head bobbing above the sink. "It must have been so hard for her to bring me up on her own."

Leo heard Stan's puffing as he shuffled back around the corner of the house followed, this time, by his dog, Winston, a Jack Russell of whom Leo was very fond. While Leo patted Winston affectionately across his back, the old man bent stiffly over the mower and removed the lead from the spark plug then handed the tool to Leo. "There, you do it. It's a bit stiff for me."

With a couple of hand jolts on the wrench Leo could feel the spark plug turning. He unscrewed it until it came loose. The young man and the old man bent over the table to inspect its insides.

"See, the points are covered with deposit; all gummed up," said Stan. "That's why it's struggling to start."

"Okay, so what now?"

"Well, we could scrape it clean, but that's not as good as putting in a new one." He stretched upright and glanced at Leo. "I suggest you pop down to the gas station; they'll have one."

Stan stood back as Leo grabbed the spark plug and bounded off to his car. "Ah, he's so full of energy. If only. . . ." He sat firmly down in a chair and waited for his breathing to calm down. "If only I had half his energy . . . how much more could be achieved."

Mandy, Leo's mother, walked out the kitchen door followed by another women unfamiliar to Stan. Winston barked at the intruder.

"Hi Stan. Where's Leo? I want to introduce him to someone."

"He's gone to get something for the lawnmower. He'll be back soon," said Stan glancing at the stranger while calling Winston over. She was a woman in her early thirties, neatly dressed and with a warm smile. "Hello."

"Oh dear, I'm being rude," said Mandy, raising her hand toward the newcomer. "This is Brenda. She's coming to live with us. She's a nurse." She raised her other hand. "And Brenda, this is Stan; he lives next door and has been our friend for many years."

"Hello Brenda; I'm assuming you're Mandy's new boarder. Good to make your acquaintance."

Stan motioned to stand up but Brenda signaled for him to remain seated, and, instead, she walked across, shook his hand, and sat in the chair next to him.

Mandy remained standing. "Good. You two get to know each other. I'll put on the kettle." She rushed off toward the kitchen.

They sat momentarily in silence while Brenda stroked Winston under his ears.

"Are you working at the local hospital?" Stan asked politely.

"Kind of," replied Brenda. "I've recently accepted a nursing job at your local hospice. I just finished my palliative care training, and this is my first permanent position. But, unfortunately, it's far from where I usually live and I'm boarding here until I can find a suitable place . . . like an apartment or a town house."

"The hospice," said Stan thoughtfully. "So you work with people who are dying?"

"Yes, that's right. I help care for their health and manage their pain, and I talk with them when they feel distressed. It's very busy work."

"You must find that emotionally draining?"

"Sometimes." Brenda glanced across and could see the old man was studying her with intense interest. "But mostly it's fairly routine. I enjoy talking with the patients, particularly about the past. They have had such interesting lives."

Mandy returned holding a tray with a pot of coffee, three mugs, and some muffins. "I baked these this morning," she stated proudly as she poured out the coffee.

"Mandy, I found out that Brenda nurses with people who are dying," stated Stan in a matter-of-fact fashion.

Mandy finished pouring the coffee, handed the mugs around and offered them milk and sugar. "That must be interesting work." She offered them each a muffin.

"Yes, I find it fascinating," replied Brenda.

Mandy sat down in a chair across the other side of the table. "So, how long does it take you to. . . ."

She was interrupted as Leo bounded around the corner of the house clutching a packet. "Here it is Stan," he declared triumphantly. He paused as he realized a stranger was present.

"Leo, this is Brenda, our new boarder," clarified Mandy.

"Hi, Brenda," he said, briefly shaking her hand then looking away. "Sorry, but we really need to get this damn thing working."

Stan hoisted himself awkwardly out of his seat and approached the mower. "Okay, you put it in, and we'll see if it starts."

Leo screwed in the sparkplug, tightened it, then reconnected the lead. He lifted the mower down to the ground, then pulled its starting cord and the engine roared immediately into action. "Great! Great, Stan. It's going!"

Stan stood for several minutes holding onto Winston's collar and watching Leo as he pushed the mower up and down the lawn. Mandy and Brenda leant close so they could hear each other over the din of the machine. Stan eventually turned and waved goodbye to the two women and headed back to his house to complete his weeding.

When Leo had finished the lawns and put the equipment away, he walked over to join Mandy and Brenda at the table.

"Thanks for doing the lawns," said Mandy. "I'll get you a nice cool drink." She stood, collected the used utensils, and headed for the kitchen.

"You're Mom's such a friendly, welcoming person," commented Brenda.

"Yes, she's nice. But she has her moments."

"You mean, getting grumpy? That's hard to imagine. But I guess we all have. . . ."

Brenda was interrupted by a single and abrupt bang on the kitchen window. They both jumped up immediately and stared around for a possible source of the sound.

"What the hell was that?" exclaimed Mandy running out of the kitchen. "Did someone throw something?"

"No, I think I saw a bird," said Brenda as she walked across to the bushes under the window. "Oh, here it is; poor thing. It's a young blackbird." She bent down and gently scooped the panting creature into her palms and carried it over to the table. Brenda opened her hands, and Mandy and Leo huddled around to assess the bird's condition. The blackbird lay without moving and without looking around. Its only movement was the quick rise and fall of its chest.

"Poor little thing," said Leo, "I think its neck's broken." He bent over and gently stroked its tiny forehead and stared into the gleaming surface of its black eyes. "So delicate and so fragile." He wondered what it might be experiencing.

The rapid rise and fall of the bird's chest slowed to an irregular pulse before ceasing altogether. The gloss in its eyes dulled, and no further movement could be detected.

Leo glanced briefly across at Brenda. She was staring down at the dead bird with an intense look of concern. "How sudden the change," commented Leo. "One moment a complex living creature, the next moment a lifeless bundle of black feathers."

These four characters will be our companions throughout the book. It will be their conversations about death that will liven up discussion and introduce varying and conflicting perspectives on the nature and meaning of my inevitable and unspeakable death.

Notes

1. Coverage of these many areas can be found in multiauthor collections of topics in death studies such as R. A. Neimeyer, ed., *Death Anxiety Handbook: Research, Instrumentation, and Application* (London: Routledge, 2015); A. Tomer, G. T. Eliason, and P. Wong, eds., *Existential and Spiritual Issues in Death Attitudes* (Mahwah: Lawrence Erlbaum, 2013).
2. As will be discussed in more detail in Chapter 2, the term "my-death" excludes interpretations of mortality that are derived from applying observations of other people's death ("other-death") to oneself.
3. Many writers on death discuss its all-pervading nature. For an overview, see B. Schumacher, *Death and Mortality in Contemporary Philosophy* (Cambridge University Press, 2010).
4. The four characters in this book are composites of features derived from the many people I have known or have worked with as either a practitioner or as a researcher. I have in no way modeled the characters on any particular individual. During the writing of the book, if I detected inadvertent resemblances to a person I have known, I have sought to water down the similarity by introducing unrelated characteristics. Accordingly, any resemblance to a particular person, whether dead or alive, is purely coincidental.

1

Other People Die

Other people die; that's what happens. Some die suddenly and unexpectedly; others die of illnesses which linger on for long periods of time.

People in general die. Newspapers will report amorphous masses of people dying from starvation, from epidemics, and from military conflicts. An article might claim that tobacco-related illnesses kill more than 480,000 people in the United States per year.[1] The numbers are so large it's difficult to get one's head around them. Sometimes these involve small groups of people, such as those dying in a bus crash or a landslide; deaths that are still shocking in their own right, particularly when those who die belong to one's own community. Sometimes those who die are unknown individuals who die in unusual circumstances, like the mother of three who fell asleep in her car and crashed into a power pole or the teenager who fell to his death base-jumping off a waterfall.

Familiar people die: leading politicians die, movie stars die, rock stars die, television personalities die. Each of their deaths leaves unnerving absences in the spaces they once occupied.

Acquaintances die; familiar people in the community cease to be around. The old man down the road was carried out from his home unceremoniously in a zipped up body bag. The woman working three offices down the corridor died unexpectedly from an aggressive brain tumor; she was the last person you'd expect to die in this manner.

Loved ones die. Oh, but this is beyond belief. A partner, a child, a parent, a lifelong friend—a loved one can be ripped away without any room for concession or negotiation. Their absence leaves a permanent hole in the fabric of daily life—so hard to accept, so hard to accommodate. The sense of violation and outrage can linger for years.

When loved ones die, their familiar fleshy bodies, so capable of expression and movement, are, in the next moment, lying stiff and immobile; their limbs drained of all energy and dynamism; a lifeless form that will never return to the living, breathing, smiling form that was so familiar before.

In these various ways, the deaths of other people swirl around us, reminding us repeatedly of the transitory nature of existence. Even as we become absorbed in the soap operas of daily life, the capacity of others to die permeates our surroundings. Perhaps, at times, this capacity becomes over-familiar and taken for granted; it warrants little consideration. Perhaps, at other times, particularly with loved ones, the capacity is something to avoid thinking about lest we become paralyzed by the fear it elicits. But its constant presence at so many levels, plus the potential for people we love to die, significantly disrupts daily life, making it difficult to completely ignore its presence.

And because each of us is still alive—none of us has died yet—what we learn about death is almost entirely derived from what we observe about the death of others. However, intertwined into these observations lies one logical consequence with complex implications. This is not an observation but a resulting idea. In every case, for every form of life ever observed, to be alive means having the capacity to die.

How did we begin to apply observations of other people's mortality to the idea of our own mortality? How did such an idea emerge during our childhoods? How does it shift and change during the course of our lives? What does it mean as we approach the end of our lives? These questions are what the following chapter intends to tackle.

Growing up with Death

Children grow up in a world pervaded by the death of other people, but, for the very early years, its presence is eclipsed by other developmental tasks such as adaptation to the complexity and wonder of life. But, slowly, observations of impermanence mount up: heroes die in movies, insects die in the sink, pets die in road accidents, old people die in hospitals, and, for some children, close family members might die when they are still very young, too young to make sense of what is going on. These observations lead progressively to the conclusion that the lives of all living organisms come to an end. But how might that apply to oneself?

The manner in which children come to recognize the biological fact of personal mortality has attracted some research attention. In 1940, Sylvia Anthony published a book describing her pioneering research on developmental changes in the way children think about death.[2] She outlined how, between the ages of five and twelve, children face several important conceptual leaps in the way death is appreciated. She noted how, initially, very young children are unlikely to see death as something pertaining to themselves, but then, as they approach five, they begin to notice, perhaps in real life or perhaps in stories and other media depictions, that extraordinary events, like accidents or shootings or even the deaths of pets, can result in a living organism no longer living. This they find both fascinating and confusing, and this confusion can spark a sequence of key realizations.

Research since Anthony's early work has identified at least five conceptual leaps that typical four- to seven-year-olds need to make regarding the physical reality of death.[3] First, they need to recognize that all living things will die one day ("inevitability"). Second, they need to appreciate that when people die their bodies and minds cease to operate ("cessation"). Third, they begin to realize that once a living organism dies nothing can be done to bring that creature back to life ("irreversibility"). Fourth, they recognize that death is caused by the breakdown of bodily functions ("causality"). Some argue this realization may take the longest "as it involves the understanding of complex processes that result in the breakdown of the body's functioning."[4] And finally they recognize that death and everything it entails applies to all people and that no one can escape it ("universality").[5] This last realization is the most complex of all because this "all people" includes one's self, and coming to terms with this all-encompassing fact extends well beyond childhood.

Of course, the sequencing of these realizations will vary according the child's context and mental abilities.[6] For example, some children will encounter the death of relatives and even friends at a young age, and this can accelerate their appreciation of mortality.[7] Moreover, the different timings of these realizations can push children in a variety of directions. For example, a child who thinks of death as related to bodily deterioration but at the same time does not see death as universally inevitable could take what might seem to adults a morbid interest in the remains of dead animals. The whole idea of death in extraordinary circumstances seems fascinating while, at the same time, it might not appear applicable to his or her own circumstances.[8] However, one of the strongest influences in the way children come to appreciate death concerns the influence that culture and religion play, particularly in relation to irreversibility and cessation.[9]

Leo walked into the kitchen to see Brenda reading a book at the table. He sat down opposite her. In the back of his mind, he was intrigued by Brenda's job: What was it like to spend most of your day with people who were dying?

"Brenda, I've never seen anyone die, only animals and pets."

She put her book down and looked across at him.

"When I was younger," Leo continued, "still at primary school, I had a pet rabbit, Alfie, who I looked after. I would feed him and clean his hutch; I was very fond of him. Then one day I thought Alfie was looking a bit subdued, so I picked him up and nursed him on my knee and tried to give it some dandelion leaves; he'd usually gobble them up straight away, but he didn't even sniff the leaves. I picked him up and sat with him in my arms. Then suddenly he started having seizures and convulsing uncontrollably. I didn't know what to do. Then he went limp and he stopped breathing."

"That must have been very hard, particularly since you'd cared for him for so long."

"Yes, I was shocked. One moment Alfie was looking at me with his cute pink eyes, the next moment he was limp and lifeless. His eyes went dull, as though he'd somehow abandoned his body. . . . Is it similar when people die?"

"Yes, I often look into people's eyes as they take their last breath. Sometimes there's a long wait between breaths, but eventually they reach their last breath, their bodies go limp, and their eyes go dull, just like what happened with Alfie. . . . So, what did you do next?"

"Well, we found a nice box and made a cushion from part of a blanket, then put flowers around him. I dug a hole in the corner of the garden, then Mom and I gently placed the box in the hole as though we were laying him down to sleep. Then we said a few words about what a good rabbit Alfie had been and how much he'd enjoyed his life."

"That seems very fitting."

"But, in hindsight, I already knew death was final and that Alfie wasn't coming back . . . so why did we pretend it isn't final?"

"Perhaps because you think of him carrying on in some way; maybe in some sort of bunny heaven."

"Yes, yes, I guess that's what we were doing."

Deep within the customs and practices of most cultures are embedded metaphors, stories, and myths about life continuing on after death. For example, in Christian traditions, stories from the Bible offer a range of potent characterizations, from the image of Christ's resurrection to the continuing presence of the saints, and from discussion on the nature of eternal life to the migration of souls into heaven. Children are typically introduced to these depictions at an early age, and they provide a potent way of downplaying the irreversibility of death and selling the idea of an enduring afterlife into which the child will eventually achieve entry. But such depictions are not limited to religious contexts. For example, both the key figures in the Disney animated films *Sleeping Beauty* and *Snow White and the Seven Dwarfs* are depicted as falling asleep rather than permanently dying,[10] and, since the 1970s, an increasing number of children's books are offering different ways of thinking about death and eternity.[11]

Leo glanced across at Brenda on the other side of the table. "So where do you think parents get this urge to pretend to children that death doesn't really happen?"

"Well, wouldn't you want to protect your child from the frightening realities of death?"

"Yeah, but I wouldn't want to fill their heads with all sorts of false stories; it'd just muddle them up and lead them to distrust what adults might say to them in the future."

"But you can see it from their point of view. The idea of a permanent parting is too difficult for children to get their heads around, particularly if it means separation from the relationships they're most dependent on, namely their parents."

"I think that idea's more difficult for parents than children. Children can adjust to pretty much anything." He cradled his chin in his hands. "Besides, it wasn't just Mom who pretended life continues after death; she was also in cahoots with most other adults: teachers talked the same way, as did uncles and aunts, neighbors and shop owners, priests and ministers. . . . All adults seemed to be in on this conspiracy."

"I wouldn't say it's a conspiracy. It doesn't really do much harm. Besides which, children may not yet have the mental and emotional capacity to take on the idea of death as permanent and final, particularly when thinking about their own deaths."

"But I reckon it can be harmful because it sets up a pattern of denial. As the child grows up, they are likely to carry on with this fantasy and the idea of living forever gets embedded deep in their minds. This would then prevent them from forming a richer and more realistic understanding of death and has the potential to magnify any fear they have of death because of the distressing confusion they experience whenever they think of it." He paused and glanced across at Brenda. "And what's more, they'd then pass this fantasy idea on to their children in a self-perpetuating circle."

The question about how honest and direct to be with children about death gains more salience when deciding what to do for children facing terminal illnesses. In an early study, Barney Glaser and Anselm Strauss (1966) studied the interactions between families and professionals around the dying child and identified a common pattern of avoiding discussions about death. Myra Bluebond-Langner, in her study of situations in which children die, described a system of "mutual pretense" where both the adults involved and the dying child participate in constructing a façade of continuation by avoiding any talk of death in order to maintain socially prescribed roles such as being a nurturing parent or a caring health professional.[12] In her summary of this research, Margaret Mahon (2011) commented:

> This refusal of some parents to discuss the possibility of death with children almost seems to be magical thinking. These parents seem to believe that discussing death would make it happen, and conversely, that positive thinking will lead to a cure.[13]

Perhaps, as Leo suggested, this "mutual pretense" around the dying child is merely an extension of a broader tendency for adults to promote ways of talking that support notions of continuation that not only protect their children but also protect themselves from unpalatable possibilities.

A Lifelong Journey

The task of developing a conceptual understanding of the physical reality of death is only part of the picture, and a full appreciation is in no way complete by the end of childhood. This is particularly the case in developing a way of understanding personal mortality. Its complexities protrude in multiple ways deep into the core of how we experience emotions, spirituality, and even consciousness in general. Childhood understandings of the fact of death comprise but a first step in the ongoing maturing of a relationship which, arguably, keeps evolving throughout our lives. While steps in our appreciation of death vary considerably between different social and cultural contexts, the following will touch briefly on key aspects from adolescence through to the later phases of old age and end-of-life.

As children transition into the teenage years they take with them an appreciation of the biological reality of death plus their culturally transmitted understanding of an afterlife. These two do not speak clearly to each other. The child's acceptance of the fact of death and the idea of living forever can generate tension and confusion. Developmental psychologists Lloyd and Illene Noppe (2004) have approached these points of confusion as linked to a set of fundamental ambiguities that they saw adolescents trying to negotiate alongside other key developmental processes, such as forming a strong individual identity separate from parents and working out which values are important. They contended that

> there are certain tensions experienced by adolescents that compromise their truly mature grasp of, and ability to cope with, a more complete and mature approach to this complex phenomenon.[14]

The type of tensions and ambiguities they face include a fascination with risk-taking just when their bodies are approaching peak condition; an emerging rationality that competes with romantic ideals such as absolute commitment and eternal love; and, as already mentioned, tension between their acceptance of finality and belief in a continuing afterlife.[15] Adolescents negotiate their way through these tensions in ways that vary from strong death anxiety to apparent total indifference. What lies at the heart of these responses is recognition that engagement with death involves more than cognitive reasoning; it is also calling them to engage emotionally with the reality of death.

A key way in which adolescents connect emotionally with death is by means of available cultural and religious representations. Throughout history, a diverse range of ways of representing death have offered themselves for imaginative deployment. The possibilities are wide-ranging and have included the use of symbols and images in pictorial depictions, the use of metaphors and myths in literature and poetry, and the use of personifications in performing arts. The French historian Philippe Ariès has written extensively on the historical influences in Western cultural interpretations and practices surrounding death.[16] He traced historical links back to a wide range of forms of expression which included medieval poetry, images on sixteenth-century gravestones and epitaphs, eighteenth-century fascinations with the corpse, and nineteenth-century preoccupations with "the beautiful death." Part of his analysis focused on the various roles the macabre plays in death representations, and, following in his footsteps, a broad scholarly literature has documented widely varying beliefs and customs which include death representations at funerals, in eulogies, in memorials, in the disposal of corpses, in poetry, and in theater.[17]

Adolescents seek out cultural spaces that enable them to connect emotionally with death. In an age with diverse forms of communication, they find many spaces where this might take place, but for many the most accessible and visually stimulating images and personifications are found in movies and on the internet.

Sitting at the kitchen table, Leo was keen to press Brenda further about her thoughts on death. "As I reached my teens, I'd learned not to trust what adults had told me about death. Mostly they carried on about people living on after death in some vague place called heaven."

Brenda repeated what she said earlier. "I guess they wanted to protect you from ideas too complex for you to handle."

"Hmm, well, about that time, me and my friends became intensely interested in images of death used in movies and computer games. Several of the girls in my class got into the Twilight Saga; hah, all those vampires with love-lorn expressions, but my group gravitated towards the walking dead, you know, zombies. It was a strange obsession—one we talked about all the time."

"Ah, at that age we were into goths and emos; you know, dressing in black and obsessing about death, self-harm, and suicide." Brenda sipped her coffee thoughtfully. "Some things don't change." She glanced across at Leo. "So why the fascination with the living dead, or the undead, or whatever you call it?"

"I guess there's something intriguing about zombies. Of course, they're completely ridiculous; hordes of contagious cannibals living on after death with a single purpose of devouring those still fully living. But, looking at it another way, they reflect the absurdity of what we were dealing with. On the one hand they connect with the fatalistic pointlessness of life and death; then, on the other hand, they keep on living, but not living in the glorious, heavenly way that adults told us about, living more in a nothingness space which represents a threat to everyone who exists."

"I've never thought of zombies that way."

"See, us losing trust in what adults told us meant we needed to seek out understandings from other sources."

The zombie is but one of a long line of cultural personifications used to give meaning to death.[18] Their images echo many of the representations of mortality that have preceded them. For example, the Dance of Death, or *danse macabre,* emerged in the late Middle Ages as a way of representing the overriding power of death. The earliest image was a mural painted in 1425, at the Cemetery of the Holy Innocents in Paris, in which a king and a cardinal stand alongside two skeleton ghouls. The popularity of this depiction then spread rapidly through Europe, not only in the form of paintings but also as sculpture, poetry, live performance, and even dancing processions.[19] In each representation death was personified in the form of macabre figures, often skeletons or emaciated bodies wearing capes. They were typically accompanied by a line-up of recognizable figures from everyday life—a noble, a preacher, a squire—who carried themselves with propriety and dignity. By way of contrast the death figures were typically presented as smiling and moving about in a chaotic and unpredictable manner. As described by Elina Gertsman (2006),

> The skeletons or half-rotted corpses that wildly skip around their victims seem to be the merriest participants of the morbid show. . . . Do they, then, reflect the advice "as whan thou spekyst of a mery mater to shew a laughiyng and mery countenance?" Not at all, for they do not address merry matters but very serious ones, albeit with sarcasm and jest. . . . [T]hey speak of death and the necessity to repent . . . they urge the consideration of the inevitable end.[20]

Dancing skeletons and marching half-rotted corpses who display little regard for those precious attachments we cling onto in life resonate with modern-day vampires, ghouls, zombies, and banshees. This is a symbolic language that draws adolescents forward and speaks to them of the meaning of death and, over time, helps them anchor an emotional connection to their own mortality.

As early adolescence advances into later adolescence,[21] the inevitability of personal mortality is more solidly internalized as part of the process variously labeled as "individuation" or "leaving home."[22] The challenge then becomes one of how to stay connected with death without becoming overwhelmed by its negativity. A common, and perhaps indirect, way for later adolescents to engage with death is by indulging in various forms of risk-taking such as speeding in cars, getting intoxicated, and participating in extreme sports.[23] Stephen Lyng (2005, 2012) has labeled these activities "edgework" and describes it as

> distinguished by the special significance of critical "edges" or boundary lines negotiated in the risk-taking endeavor. At the most abstract level, the "edge" is best understood as the boundary between order and disorder, form and form-lessness . . . involving more concretely the lines separating life and death, full functionality and permanent disability, consciousness and unconsciousness, or sanity and insanity. . . . Although edgeworkers try to prepare for dangers that can be anticipated, their primary quest is to confront and manage challenges that are entirely unpredictable . . . which propels them to get as close as possible to the edge without actually crossing it.
>
> The focus on decisive boundary lines reflects at one level the corporeal nature of the "edges" negotiated in this form of risk-taking. In the archetype of edgework represented by many extreme sports, edgeworkers confront the line separating a conscious living body from an unconscious dead corpse, or some approximation of this distinction. Hence, in the death-defying forms of edgework, risk-takers use their skills to manage fixed boundaries and confrontations with these objective edges produce a sense of authentic experience.[24]

During the risk activity, edgeworkers connect to mortality in a way that involves far more than a conceptual relationship. In the midst of taking a death-defying risk, contact is being made with death in more than a concep-tual way; the connection is deeply emotional and existentially significant.[25]

The early adult years are often given over to affairs of the world: earning a living, establishing a career, entering sexual partnerships, and having chil-dren. It is also typically a period of good health and vitality, a time when personal mortality can seem a long way in the distance. However, while the pressure of establishing an adult identity often squeezes out concerns about mortality, the reality of death still extends its hand out to touch various aspects of life.

After Leo returned to study in his bedroom, Brenda wandered into the lounge where Mandy was relaxing in front of television.

"Ah, Brenda," greeted Mandy, as she pointed the television's remote to lower the volume. "I could hear you and Leo chatting. What were you discussing?"

Brenda sat down in the armchair by the fireplace. She felt a little annoyed at Mandy's direct questioning. She also recognized that she needed to answer her carefully. "He was talking about his enjoyment of zombie movies, and I was telling him about my being a goth."

"Ah, his morbid interests again. When will he focus on the more positive things?"

"I don't know. Perhaps it's a phase he needs to work through," said Brenda, still annoyed at being cross-questioned. "What about you Mandy? Weren't there times you felt drawn by images of death."

"Mostly no; I try not to think about it." She had detected the annoyance in Brenda's tone so she allowed their conversation to stall into silence. "Ah, actually, there was a time that I found myself thinking about death." She paused again. "You know, Brenda, having a child changes everything. When I was pregnant with Leo, I remember being troubled by so many thoughts and fears about him dying. Then, as the birth approached, I also worried about my own death."

"Yes, I guess the moment a child is born, you are forever tied to the possibility of its death."

"Yes, but it's more than that. When Leo was born, my death mattered for a different reason. There lay this baby; so vulnerable, so needy, so dependent on me; I knew this reliance was going to continue for decades. Imagine if I was to die; he would not be able to survive, or, at least, survive in the same way. So the threat that I might die became a profound threat to the child. I wasn't scared for me, but scared for him."

Even in the midst of the busyness of early adulthood, with death far away on the horizon, the specter of death still manages to reach out and make contact during special private moments, perhaps passing in moments of anxiety, of confusion, of reflection, and, sometimes, of awe.

Midlife, which stretches imprecisely between the ages of forty and sixty, is a period when a number of important transitions occur leading into old age. These transitions typically include children leaving home, the stabilization of home and work life, and preparations for retirement. But perhaps the most notable change has to do with perceptions regarding the proximity of one's own death. During the early adult years death is likely to be seen as an event far off in the future, something that happens to other people—mainly older people—and seen as so distant it is hardly worth worrying about. By contrast, in midlife, a variety of changes begin to signal how death is not as far away as previously expected. Many of these signals originate from the aging body: changes in appearance—such as balding and wrinkles—changes in strength and dexterity and the onset of chronic medical conditions, such as arthritis, chronic back pain, diabetes, and hearing difficulties. While actual time until death proceeds at a steady rate, perceptions and expectations regarding this span of time can be highly elastic.[26] For example, a man in his midlife who, through most his adulthood, had thought little about my-death, might begin to notice decreases in his general agility, and, in response, he might suddenly see his death as approaching worryingly fast; from way in the distance, it now seems to be hurtling toward him, compressing his future into a narrow time horizon. His response to this might be exaggerated. Perhaps as a result of years of ignoring death, it is suddenly seen as much closer than would be realistic to expect. Over time his perceptions might become more realistic, but, on occasions when he does see it as closing in, this then prompts a series of questions: Where did all that time go? What have I achieved with my life? And why can't I have another go?

In popular parlance such moments of reflection and life re-evaluation are commonly referred to as a "midlife crisis." Some writers have described in detail the main ingredients of such crises.[27] For example, the Canadian psychoanalyst Elliott Jaques (1965) characterized a midlife crisis as follows:

> *The simple fact of the situation is the arrival at the mid-point of life. What is simple from the point of view of chronology, however, is not simple psychologically. The individual has stopped growing up, and has begun to grow old. . . . The achievement of mature and independent adulthood presents itself as the main psychological task. The paradox is that of entering the prime of life, the stage of fulfilment, but at the same time the prime and fulfilment are dated. Death lies beyond.[28]*

But now, more than fifty years on, little evidence can be found to support the idea of a definitive stage understood as a midlife crisis. If it was a significant "crisis," then midlife would show more signs of challenges to psychological well-being than occurs in other life phases, and that, according to research, has simply not been found to be the case.[29] Alternatively, Alexandra Freund and Johannes Ritter (2009) have proposed placing the idea of a definitive "crisis" to one side and focusing instead on midlife as a transition phase involving "challenges to life management."

Due to strong social expectations that middle adulthood is a time for reviewing one's accomplishments, people are more likely to compare their actual self-image with their ideal self-image as well as with social expectations of what one ought to have achieved by middle adulthood. Moreover, because middle adulthood is commonly viewed as the middle of life, the change in future time perspective as the time until death is likely to highlight the limited remaining time for redirecting or correcting one's personal developmental path.[30]

So, following their suggestion, increased awareness of the constraints and limitations imposed by age and appreciation of the relentless approach of death can be seen as prompting periods of re-evaluation leading to a refocusing of values, commitments, and decisions on how the remainder of life will be pursued.[31] Many aspects of these periods will be discussed later in the book, particularly when the critical role of finitude will be examined in Chapters 6 and 7.

By old age, signals of approaching death tend to arrive thick and fast. The markers of a deteriorating body, first identified in midlife, multiply and become more intense. It might start with unwanted changes in appearance—such as sagging skin or a stooped posture—then progress to changes in functionality—difficulties opening jars or managing stairs—then move on to affecting mobility—not being able to drive or difficulties walking. Added to this are steady increases in exposures to death. Parents have probably already passed away, but now friends and other contemporaries, including siblings and cousins, begin to die with worrying regularity, and attending funerals becomes a routine event. On top of this are the periods spent in hospitals and rest homes where, again, the deaths of acquaintances and friends in adjacent beds or next rooms reinforce awareness of the unmistakable reality of one's approaching death. This equips older people with a strong and accurate sense of their proximity to death. For example, Dana Kotter-Grühn and colleagues (2010) used data from a Berlin longitudinal study to show how older people have a surprisingly accurate idea of how close they are to death.[32]

Despite continuing to fear death and despite strong individual differences, older people are still able to move forward into a manageable relationship with their mortality. For example, Monika Ardelt (2013) recruited 164 older people in the United States living in a mixture of settings, including their own homes, rest homes, and hospices, and asked them to complete a battery of questionnaires focused on attitudes toward death, religious orientation, purpose in life, and measures of what she called "wisdom." Among her findings were two interesting observations: first, that being afraid of death did not appear related to accepting death and, second, that neither wisdom nor a sense of purpose in life appeared to be required in accepting death. Ardelt explained these results by pointing out that since older people have more exposures to the death of other people,

> [they] might have come to terms with the finitude of their life and might even look forward to a life after death and a reunion with the loved ones, while still being afraid of the unknown that death represents. Other older adults might be neither afraid of death nor avoid thinking about it, but they also might not be convinced that there is indeed a life after death. In fact, the relation between belief in an afterlife and death anxiety is not clear.[33]

This also suggests that a person's relationship to death in old age is dynamic and capable of including many moments of deliberation and multiple shifts in perspective.

The waning strength of an aging body culminates, for most, in the end-of-life phase, a period of variable duration when it is clear that death is approaching and when preparations for leaving are put in place. Aspects of this phase will be discussed in more detail in Chapter 11, but one aspect concerns the close relationship that can developed between someone dying and a person caring for them.

> Mandy looked up from the magazine she was browsing and gazed across at Brenda who was still sitting in the armchair totally immersed in a book she was reading. "Brenda, I don't know how you can spend your whole day with people who are dying. You must find it very depressing."
>
> Brenda looked up and adjusted her focus. "No, I wouldn't work in the area if I felt that way. Mostly, I feel very positive about my work because I know I'm really helping people, both people who're dying and their families."
>
> "But you're constantly forming relationships that don't last. You know they won't be around for long. Don't you find it hard to form close ties only to lose them a few weeks later?"
>
> "Yeah, that can be a challenge. As a nurse, you do get very close to those you care for, particularly when they're finding things distressing. And some people really do feel miserable and desperate right to the end."

"Yes, that's how I'd find it; terrifying. There surely can't be any joy in sitting there waiting to meet your maker."

"Yes, but that only applies to a few people. I have nursed others who do anything but wait to die. They might start out initially shocked and confused, but during the course of their care they somehow manage to make really big changes in how they engage with their dying process. Poised there at the edge of death they can make changes very fast, moving quickly through a big range of emotions—fear, anger, guilt, even excitement and joy—and making large leaps in the way they talk about death. At one point they might see death as some form of enemy besieging them and attacking them from the outside, then at another point death becomes some sort of friend talking to them quietly and beckoning them forward. I'm just amazed at how many different ways they experience death and at the number of people who seem to manage somehow to reach a point of peace and reconciliation."

"I'm glad to hear that," said Mandy, pausing to ponder on what she'd heard, then, speaking slowly, she asked. "I guess that allows you to gain a sense of what it might be like to die?"

"I get a chance to see the wide range of possible ways of facing death, but it provides me little sense of how I would handle it when my time comes."

End of life is another leg of our journey alongside death as we advance through life. As a social context it offers those who participate, particularly those who care for the dying, a special opportunity to appreciate the complex physical, mental, emotional, and spiritual dimensions in their own relationship to death.

Applying It to One's Self

To summarize key points in this chapter, the bulk of what we know about death comes from observing the death of others. From these observations we work out that death is inevitable and universal, we see that it involves the body ceasing to function, we see that it entails being separated from the people we love, we see that it can be painful and upsetting, and we can empathize with how it might feel to find out when one is going to die. Overlaying what we learn from the death of others is the possibility of losing a loved one. This can occur at any stage—childhood, adolescence, midlife, and old age—and can have the effect of magnifying and sometimes accelerating what is being learned at each stage. As mentioned earlier, the death of a seven-year-old child's mother can have the effect of accelerating the child's cognitive understanding of the physical reality of death. Similarly, the adolescent who loses a sibling is more quickly confronted by the emotional significance of death. The loss of a loving partner during adulthood or midlife allows death to step across the threshold right into the heart of the home; for adults, this encourages them to reflect on death, and, for those in their midlife, it can trigger profound existential questioning that can lead to a re-evaluation of what they want out of life. As old age progresses, more and more friends and family pass away, but the loss of someone very close can still hit hard, with the potential of unleashing the full potency of one's approaching mortality.

Threaded as a continuous strand among what we learn about death is what we glean specifically about personal mortality. The two faces of death, other-death and my-death, are tangled up together and it is not always clear which of the two is being referenced. During middle childhood the inevitability of death is gradually seen as applying to all people, but this "all people" could be seen as applying to both other people and to one's self. In adolescence emotional engagement via cultural images and symbols of death might be read as referring both to death in general and to the death of other people, but they can equally be referring to one's own death. For example, the image of a skeleton on a poster can be read as referring to the skeletons of other people, but it can also be viewed as though one's own skeleton is smiling back. During midlife and old age, the looming presence of death certainly heightens awareness of personal mortality, but this is interwoven with other aspects such as a fear of aging, anticipated loss of other loved ones, and fears regarding the process of dying.

Arriving home from work, Brenda parked her car by the footpath outside the house, clambered out, opened the trunk, and pulled out two bags of groceries with ingredients for dinner. As she turned toward the gate she noticed Stan checking his letterbox.

"Hi Stan. Had a good day?" She walked across and placed the groceries down next to the fence.

"Ah, Brenda. Yes, the weather's been fine, and I've been weeding my lettuces." He walked across to stand on the other side of the fence. "I suppose you've had a long day listening to the dying?"

"Yep, that's right," she nodded. "It was a fairly emotionally up-and-down sort of day." She paused for a few moments and ran her fingers along the top of the fence. "It's funny Stan, both Mandy and Leo have been asking me about my job; they keep questioning me about how I find it. One's fascinated, the other's horrified. And I'm not quite sure what either of them is after."

"Well, I guess because you work all week with the dying, they think you've got stronger insights than other people."

"It may seem like that, but I'm not sure I do." Brenda picked up her groceries. "I think Mandy is asking me because she wants to understand more about other people's death. But I think with Leo . . . I think he's hovering around some sort of change in how he looks at death. Neither of them, I think, is quite sure why they're interested. Maybe it's curiosity, maybe it's morbid fascination, or maybe it's something deeper."

"Hmm," said Stan as he bent over to stroke Winston, who had been nudging his legs. "Do you think they might be chasing the same thing? I mean, death is death, whether it's to do with me or to do with another person, it's pretty much the same thing."

"I've wondered that, too," said Brenda as she motioned to walk away. "No, I reckon they're responding at different levels; Mandy's concerns with other people's death are rooted in something completely different from Leo's concerns about his own death."

Here lies the principal mission for this book. It is attempting to tease out the strand of personal mortality from its confused entanglement with other aspects of death, such as the process of dying, the death of other people, and death's representation in concepts and images.[34]

Notes

1. US Department of Health and Human Services, *The Health Consequences of Smoking—50 Years of Progress: A Report of the Surgeon General* (Atlanta: US Department of Health and Human Services, 2014).

2. S. Anthony, *The Child's Discovery of Death: A Study in Child Psychology* (Abingdon Oxon: Routledge, 2013, 1940). Also see, M. Nagy, "The child's theories concerning death," *Journal of Genetic Psychology* (73, 3–27, 1948) who was at the same time researching age-related changes in understandings of death.

3. See this summarized in V. Slaughter and M. Griffiths, "Death understanding and fear of death in young children," *Clinical Child Psychology and Psychiatry* (12:4, 525–35, 2007).

4. G. Panagiotaki et al., "British and Pakistani children's understanding of death: Cultural and developmental influences," *British Journal of Developmental Psychology* (33:1, 31–44, 2015) p. 32.

5. A summary of the research literature on this is provided in T. A. Gavrilova, "The problem of children's understanding of death," *Psychological Science and Education* (4, online, 2009).

6. A summary of many aspects of children's conceptions of death is provided by B. L. Kenyon, "Current research in children's conceptions of death," *Omega: Journal of Death and Dying* (43:1, 63–91, 2001). Also see C. R. Cotton and L. Range, "Children's death concepts," *Journal of Clinical Child Psychology* (19:2, 123–27, 1990).

7. S. M. Jay et al. reported on accelerations in conceptual understandings of death following death of a close relative in "Differences in death concepts between children with cancer and physically healthy children," *Journal of Clinical Child Psychology* (16:4, 301–06, 1987).

8. A good summary of the literature is provided in a PhD thesis by M. Hopkins, "*The Development of Children's Understanding of Death*" (University of East Anglia, 2014).

9. Considerable research has been conducted in this area. See S. Brent and M. Speece, "'Adult' conceptualization of irreversibility," *Death Studies* (17:3, 203–34, 1993), and S. Yang and S. Chen, "Content analysis of free-response narratives to personal meanings of death among Chinese children and adolescents," *Death Studies* (30:3, 217–41, 2006).

10. While acknowledging this happened in Disney films prior to the 1970s, in their analysis of twenty-three Disney films, M. Cox, E. Garrett and J. Graham, "Death in Disney films," *Omega: Journal of Death and Dying* (50:4, 267–80, 2005) found they mostly depicted death as permanent and worthy of mourning, particularly when the heroes in the films died.

11. See D. Poling and J. Hupp, "Death sentences: A content analysis of children's death literature," *The Journal of Genetic Psychology* (169:2, 165–76, 2008).

12. See M. Bluebond-Langner, *The Private Worlds of Dying Children* (Princeton, NJ: Princeton University Press, 1978).

13. Quote in M. Mahon, "Death in the lives of children," in V. Talwar, P. Harris, and M. Schleifer, eds., *Children's Understanding of Death* (Cambridge: Cambridge University Press, 2011) p. 68.

14. L. Noppe and I. Noppe, "Ambiguity in adolescent understandings of death," in C. Corr and D. Balk, eds., *Handbook of Adolescent Death and Bereavement* (New York: Springer, 2004) p. 25.

15. I. Noppe and L. Noppe, "Adolescent experiences with death: Letting go of immortality," *Journal of Mental Health Counseling* (26:2, 146–67, 2004).

16. Philippe Ariès presents his thinking on the cultural dimensions of death in two major books, *Western Attitudes Toward Death: From the Middle Ages to the Present* (Baltimore: Johns Hopkins University Press, 1974) and *The Hour of Our Death* (New York: Knopf, 1981).

17. For example, an edited collection by D. Irish et al., eds., *Ethnic Variations in Dying, Death and Grief* (Philadelphia: Taylor & Francis, 2014), details many of the differences in death customs among a broad range of cultures.

18. The rise of the zombies is outlined in K. Bishop, *American Zombie Gothic: The Rise and Fall (and Rise) of the Walking Dead in Popular Culture* (Jefferson: McFarland, 2011)

and in a collection by S. McIntosh and M. Leverette, eds., *Zombie Culture: Autopsies of the Living Dead* (Lanham: Scarecrow Press, 2008).

19. These are described by E. Gertsman, "Pleyinge and peyntynge: Performing the dance of death," *Studies in Iconography* (27, 1–43, 2006).

20. Ibid., p. 17.

21. In their overview of adolescence and death, D. Balk and C. Corr, "Adolescents, developmental tasks and encounters with death and bereavement," in C. Corr and D. Balk, eds., *Handbook of Adolescent Death and Bereavement* (New York: Springer, 2004; pp. 3–24), break adolescence into three subperiods—early, middle, late—each with its own conceptual dynamics with death.

22. An overview of these processes is provided in S. Koepke and J. Denissen, "Dynamics of identity development and separation–individuation in parent–child relationships during adolescence and emerging adulthood," *Developmental Review* (32:1, 67–88, 2012).

23. Theories on adolescent risk-taking are summarized by J. Arnett, "Reckless behavior in adolescence," *Developmental Review* (12:4, 339–73, 1992).

24. S. Lyng, "Existential transcendence in late modernity: Edgework and hermeneutic reflexivity," *Human Studies* (35:3 401–14, 2012) p. 410.

25. See S. Lyng, "Sociology at the edge: Social theory and voluntary risk taking," in his *Edgework: The Sociology of Risk Taking* (New York: Routledge, 2005).

26. In an early study, L. Dickstein and S. Blatt, "Death concern, futurity, and anticipation," *Journal of Consulting Psychology* (30:1, 11–17, 1966) introduced the concept of "futurity" as the time a person expected to live and then explored how intelligence and other variables might affect it.

27. For a summary of developmental literature on midlife, see U. Staudinger and S. Bluck, "A view on midlife development from life-span theory," in M. Lachman, ed., *Handbook of Midlife Development* (Hoboken: Wiley, 2001; pp. 3–39).

28. E. Jaques, "Death and the mid-life crisis," *International Journal of Psycho-Analysis* (46:4, 502–14, 1965) p. 506.

29. See a summary of this critique in J. Reid and S. Willis, "Middle age," in S. Willis and J. Reid, eds., *Life in the Middle: Psychological and Social Development in Middle Age* (San Diego: Academic Press, 1999; pp. 276–80).

30. A. Freund and J. Ritter, "Midlife crisis: A debate," *Gerontology* (55:5, 582–91, 2009) p. 589.

31. J. Osborne, "An existential perspective on death anxiety, retirement, and related research problems," *Canadian Journal of Aging* (36:2, 246–55, 2017).

32. D. Kotter-Grühn et al., "Predicting one's own death," *European Journal of Ageing* (7:4, 293–300, 2010), explored perceptions of nearness to death in those older than seventy years and found surprising accuracy in their perceptions.

33. M. Ardelt, "Wisdom, religiosity, purpose in life, and death attitudes of aging adults," in A. Tomer et al., eds., *Existential and Spiritual Issues in Death Attitudes* (Mahwah: Lawrence Erlbaum, 2013) p. 151.

34. J. Lizza, *Persons, Humanity and the Definition of Death* (Baltimore: John Hopkins University Press, 2005) explores the complexities of death that go beyond death as a biological event.

2

My-Death

Other-death in its various guises happens in the midst of everyday life and can be referred to and discussed. My-death functions at a different level and is less easy to pinpoint or talk about. Peter Koestenbaum (1971) focused on this contrast by highlighting the significant difference between what he called "death of self" and "death of another":

> ... if a man examines closely ... what it means of another person [to die], he recognizes that he himself is still in the picture: he is the observer contemplating the scene, even if the scene is only in his imagination. Death is an event in the world, while the life-world—the world of human experience—perdures.
>
> The situation is altogether different if we subject the conception of my own death. ... Our own death means the total disintegration and dissolution of our personal worlds.[1]

When other people die, I am able to observe what is going on as it unfolds and then to observe what happens afterward. Because I witness what happens next, I am able to interpret other people's dying as an absence of what had previously existed. At one time they were living, breathing, interacting, and communicating, and the next moment they are no longer there; against the backdrop of all that remains, they have turned into an absence. When it comes to my own death, this vantage point from which I observe death as an absence no longer applies. My-death throws up the possibility of the end of my consciousness. This finality places at risk the whole notion of a continuing world; the backdrop, as it were, is under threat. Thinking of it as an absence only makes sense when it is contrasted with some form of continuity. My-death threatens this continuity and thereby disrupts applications of what we know about other-death to make sense of my-death.[2]

This chapter sets out to look more closely at the challenges we face in moving from an other-death perspective to a my-death perspective. It peers into the experiences of our four characters as a way of exploring, first, the attractions of thinking about death in terms of other-death, then to outline some of the problems and complications that follow from this perspective, and it will finish with an alternative view of my-death as understood in terms of global annihilation.

The Transposed Observer

The application of what we know from the death of others in order to make sense of our own deaths involves imagining ourselves as inhabiting the experience of another person as they die and perhaps as they move forward into some form of afterlife. There are many aspects to how we transpose the reality of someone else's death onto our individual existence. A key trigger can be news about the death of a close friend or relative or someone with whom we might identify.[3]

Mandy knocked gently on Leo's partly opened bedroom door.

Leo looked up from his computer. "It's okay, come on in."

She walked carefully across the bedroom and perched on the edge of his bed and waited for him to exit his computer.

He swiveled his chair around, "So, what's up?"

"Um, well, I have some sad news." She paused to watch a concerned look spread across his face. Best not to delay news like this too long. She plunged into what she had intended to say. "Aunty Sue passed away last night."

His initial look of surprise turned quickly into one of confusion. This was the first time anyone he actually knew, and knew well, had died. Several years earlier a boy in a class below him, Jason, had died along with his father in a head-on traffic accident. Everyone was shocked and saddened by this extraordinary event. Leo, like everyone else, thought it was unbelievably tragic that someone so young had had his life cut short. He remembered how he shuddered when he thought of such an event happening to himself.

But the boy's death was different from Aunty Sue's. He was just someone he'd played with occasionally, but Aunty Sue was someone he had spent a great deal of time with, seeing her sometimes as much as once a week, and this stretched back as far as he could remember. They often went out together to parks or movies and sometimes went on holidays together. No, Aunty Sue's departure had far more consequences than the boy at school.

"When did it happen?" he asked, not knowing what else to say.

"Someone found her in her bed this morning around ten. Luckily an old friend had dropped by to take her shopping. She must have passed away in the middle of the night. She had been. . . ."

Mandy's voice trailed off into the background. An image of Aunty Sue was forming in his mind. She was carrying a mug of hot chocolate into her bedroom and placing it on the side table next to her bed. She eased herself into the bed and propped her back up with the pillow. She slowly sipped her hot chocolate while staring at and occasionally turning the pages of her crime novel. When tiredness seemed to be coming on, she put her mug and book to one side, switched off her bedside lamp, then turned over into the darkness of her pillow.

Then, maybe, sometime in the middle of the night, she had woken up with shooting pains in her chest. She had tried to sit up but the pain was overwhelming, and, as panic spread, she was having difficulty breathing. More panic; her arms were thrashing; she could no longer breathe, and then . . . and then everything went blank . . . an absolute blankness . . . a permanent blankness.

Leo stared fiercely across at Mandy with an expression of absolute horror.

"I know, I know," reassured Mandy, "It's a terrible loss."

Leo's regular contact with Aunty Sue had enabled him to construct an understanding of how she was likely to be experiencing events at any one particular point in time. Of course he was not able to stare directly into her consciousness and observe what was going on, but, based on the many intense moments he had shared with her and from observing what she had to say and its congruence with her many changes in posture and expression, he was confident that he had a fairly accurate picture of what she was experiencing.[4] This empathic understanding formed the basis for him to identify with her inner world and then to project himself onto how he imagined she might have experienced her dying.

The empathic appreciation of the death of someone close enables us to form an understanding of what it might be like to die. For many this can be strengthened through opportunities for contact with people who are in the process of dying.[5] Exposure to people dying also elicits a wide range of emotional responses, including grief and anguish—strong emotions which can eclipse reflections on the nature of one's own mortality.[6] Indeed, some of those in regular contact with the dying may struggle with opening up to such empathic connections and might even seek ways of mentally protecting themselves from what they are encountering.[7] Nonetheless, the stark reality of losing a loved one does have the capacity to interrupt the flow of normal living and to prompt some thoughts about my-death.

Leo was walking home from the bus station, his mind absorbed by the upsetting events of the last few days. As he approached his home, he nodded to Stan who was busy pulling weeds out of his front garden.

Stan stretched stiffly upright and smiled kindly. "I'm sorry to hear about your Aunt."

"Aunty Sue, yeah, thanks, that's all right."

The old man paused and examined the pained expression across the young man's face. "Come on in. Come and join me in a cup of tea. I've got something to show you."

Leo followed him up the path and around the side of the house to the back door from where they moved from the kitchen into the lounge. Stan pulled out an old photo album from a chest in the corner of the room and sat down on the couch next to Leo. "There, that's the two of you; your Aunty Sue and you, at around four years old."

"Goodness. She's so young . . . Quite good-looking . . . I can't remember her like that."

"Yes, she certainly attracted her share of male attention."

"Funny how she never married?"

"That didn't stop her having lots of relationships," stated Stan with a twinkle in his eye.

"It's hard to imagine someone like that; so young, so vibrant . . . so much alive. Now. . . ."

They both sat in silence staring down at the photo on Stan's lap.

Then, almost in a whisper, Leo said, "I guess that's where life leads. We all have to die eventually."

Stan turned his head to face Leo. "Now, what do you mean by 'we all have to die eventually?'" He raised his eyebrows quizzically. "Sounds to me like you're trying to tell me something."

"No, no, I'm not referring to you," clarified Leo, "I was thinking of myself. I was just making the point that it's inevitable for all of us. No one escapes. And that's that, pure and simple."

Leo and Stan concurred that death is both an inevitable and inescapable consequence of being alive. But there was something in this that stretched out beyond an observation of the reality or the fact of personal mortality. Leo's "that's that" signaled something more; as though the fact carried with it layer upon layer of additional significance.

"You make it sound so simple, so matter of fact," said Stan as he placed the photo album back in the chest. "But, really, the inevitability of our death is not really a simple matter." He sat back on the couch. "As you know, I spent several years serving in Vietnam, and every day we were reminded about this inevitability when we heard of the deaths of fellow soldiers. We all had our different ways of coping with it: some, like you, just said, 'It'll come when it comes.' Others worried continuously because they constantly saw the inevitable around the next corner. Others, like myself, imagined we were in a special category and that the inevitable was something that happened to other people."

"Hmm," said Leo, "so, you're saying the fact of inevitability matters less than how we interpret it?"

"Yes. When it comes to the inevitability of death there are just so many different ways it can be understood."

"But that doesn't change the reality of each of us dying. I can spin it in different ways, but the reality doesn't change."

"Ahh, but I think the reality and the interpretation are mixed up together," said Stan staring out of the window. "Look, I'll give you another example: I remember when a cousin living in France died of lung cancer, and then the urn with her ashes was brought back home for a memorial service. After the ceremony, outside the church, I saw another cousin and the dead cousin's sister walking with the urn down a side street. They looked like they wanted to unwind; they were chatting and smoking, but—and this surprised me—as they smoked they dabbed the ash from the end of their cigarettes into the urn."

"Oooh, that's macabre," grimaced Leo. "It's almost sacrilegious."

"That was my first reaction. But then I thought about it a bit more. My cousin had been a heavy smoker from a young girl, so lung cancer was on the cards. She had her first serious bout of cancer ten years earlier from which, against all odds, she managed to survive. Then, after her recovery, she continued to smoke."

"That's remarkable. She must have been really hooked on nicotine."

"I think the sister was acknowledging something. She saw me and smiled, but her and her cousin weren't laughing, and they showed no embarrassment. It seemed to me they were, in their own way, completing the ceremony by recognizing a basic aspect of my cousin's life; her powerful relationship to tobacco. It was an important part of who she was, and it represented something significant about her mortal being."

"You mean, her smoking represented her death?"

"I guess, in a way, it signaled something about the inevitability of her death as well as the inevitability of her relationship to tobacco."

Stan was pointing out how ongoing exposure to the threat of dying, whether that involves fighting in war zones or struggling with a life-threatening disease, introduces new layers of meaning and significance regarding my-death.[8]

Abiding Observers

Other-death perspectives, so far, have relied on our ability to imagine ourselves into the experience of another person, most likely someone very close, but there is another aspect to this maneuver. If we can manage this for one person, we can also manage it with more than one person. Through a series of empathic reconstructions of other people's death, we are able to build up a sense of a collective of people who have experienced death and then to imagine them as congregating at some abiding vantage point that enables ongoing observation of everyday life below. In this way, when someone close dies, they can be understood to be joining others on this observation post, almost as though it is some eternally established platform for enduring and benevolent surveillance.

Mandy drove her car into the carpark of the funeral home. She turned off the engine, glanced sideways at Leo, then returned to staring out the window. They both sat silently for a few moments.

"Okay, well, let's get this over and done with," said Mandy nervously as she opened the car door.

They walked into the waiting room close to the main entrance. Mandy sat down on a faded armchair and flipped nervously through a magazine. The funeral home assistant entered and beckoned them to follow him down the hall. He led them through into a small carpeted room surrounded by shelves with plastic flowers. In the center of the room stood a coffin with its lid on. The assistant pulled up two chairs close to the coffin and gestured for them to sit down, then he gently raised the coffin lid to reveal Aunty Sue.

Leo could hear a faint draw-back of breath from his mother as she gazed down at her sister. Initially he was worried about how she'd handle the situation but, to his surprise, she drew her chair quietly forward, leant over and gently clasped one of her sister's hands. There she sat leaning forward, motionless and expressionless, staring at her sister's stiff smile.

Leo stood up and bent over next to his mother and gazed down at Aunty Sue's lifeless body. She lay incongruously still and looked considerably thinner than he remembered. Her face seemed slightly unreal, as though it was a wax model from Madame Tussaud's. He lowered his hand and gently stroked her cheek. It didn't feel like wax; her skin was cool and silky.

He sat back on his seat to observe the scene. He began thinking about the many other bodies that must have lain in coffins in this very same spot. Other families would have huddled around talking to, staring at, and touching their loved-one's body just as they were doing. He imagined the many souls belonging to these bodies congregating in some dimension or some place and somehow being able to watch the grief of their loved ones. They, too, would like to reach out and stroke the faces of their loved ones and to quietly utter consoling words. But such things are not possible. The worlds have been permanently split apart.

His thoughts were interrupted by a barely audible sob from Mandy. He leaned forward and laid his hand on her shoulder. She sat up abruptly.

"I think it's time to go," she said. "We need to work out what we're going to say at the funeral."

Leo had realized that transposing his consciousness empathically into his aunt's experience of death would not work if it was only applied to her. For there to be some form of continuation, some form of afterlife, this process would need to be somehow already established; it would be strange if it were to begin only with her. What would make more sense would be an afterlife that had been established from the beginning of time and that included those who had died so far.[9] Leo's aunt's point of death, thought of in this way, could be interpreted not only as a transition, but also as a process of joining an already established group of abiding observers.

The idea of life continuing after death has found expression in a wide range of philosophical and religious traditions including those belonging to Chinese, Middle Eastern, and European civilizations.[10] Central to these has been the idea of a special place for deceased souls to go to after death, a place generally referred to as "heaven." The Judo-Christian version of heaven emerged over long periods and was heavily influenced by concepts from ancient Egyptian and Mesopotamian civilizations.[11] Our inheritance of heaven into modern times is best characterized as layered and fluid. Some may think of it as a place, but equally it can be thought of as not occupying time or space. It can be seen as somewhere specifically for people who have lived good or virtuous lives, but, at the same time, it can be seen as a place for all comers. It can also be imagined as a location with specific appealing features—perhaps cushioned in the clouds, perhaps in a garden, perhaps in a beautiful building—but equally it can be thought of as a dimensional plane devoid of any familiar features.[12]

Leo and Mandy entered the small white church that sat in chocolate-box fashion between a green field and a graveyard strewn with mossy headstones. It was the same church which Aunty Sue had regularly attended on Sunday mornings. A few family friends, some distant relatives, and a handful of parishioners were sitting in scattered bunches along the pews, whispering as they awaited the ceremony. Aunty Sue's darkly varnished coffin had been placed on a shiny metal trolley and stood alone before the stairs that rose up to the altar.

The minister began by praising Aunty Sue for her simple, honest life and her devotion to faith and family. He talked of her moving on from this mortal life to another eternal life in heaven; a life bathed in the grace of God.

Leo stared down at his shoes and recalled the happy times they had had on holiday together. The times when they walked over the hills during the day and played cards late into the night. . . .

It was reassuring to think of Aunty Sue's existence persisting some-where else; somewhere surrounded by others who have departed and who together were looking down on him. Heaven would be as good a place as any: perhaps she would still play the occasional card game; perhaps she is up there now looking down on this ceremony, smiling gently at what the minister is saying; perhaps her soul is even able to stare directly into his mind, reading his feelings and his motives. Perhaps in the future she would be sitting up above and continuing to watch over him, checking out how he is managing; perhaps sending subtle messages of support during difficult times.

Leo was making use of the image of heaven as an idealized place, an ethereal realm, where aspects of Aunty Sue persisted with others in some form of ongoing continuation. At this difficult time, the notion of Aunty Sue's soul persisting in another place or dimension enabled him to view her death as a point of transition rather than as an abrupt ending. He also found it comforting how, just as her soul was reuniting with others who had died, so it followed that his soul would eventually be reuniting with her soul when his own death forced his soul to leave his body. Aunty Sue's individualized self may have departed, but her presence in an ongoing relationship could still be maintained because her spiritual essence, her soul-minus-her-body, still persisted in a domain, or some other dimension, where other souls endured.

On the flipside of seeing death as a transition point to the community of abiding observers is seeing death as the point at which we depart from our current social world, departing particularly from those who really care about us. This provides a further opportunity for looking at my-death in terms of other-death.

> The minister voice droned rhythmically as he recited some prayers. Leo gazed across at Aunty Sue's coffin. He visualized her frail old body lying peacefully inside the box, her lips spread slightly apart in an enigmatic smile. Perhaps a small crack in the lid would allow some light to penetrate thereby enabling her to see the smooth white satin lining covering the inside of her coffin? Perhaps she could hear the faint murmur of the minister's voice? Perhaps she could smell the bouquet of flowers on the lid? Perhaps her body is now relinquishing her spirit? Perhaps. . . .
>
> Leo's thoughts meandered aimlessly: Aunty Sue is in this strange box at the bottom of the altar steps. The presence of the box announces her departure. But, ah, she was a good person; far more than an Aunty: a regular companion, a friend, a soul mate. It will be so difficult not having her around. It will take them a long time to adapt to her absence.
>
> Leo felt pressure welling up behind his eyes, and he fought to prevent tears or sobs. He wiped his eyes as though they were itchy. He felt a panicky fear that his subtle weeping might escalate into more conspicuous crying so he sought to suppress it by thinking of other things.
>
> His mind finally settled on what it might be like when he himself finally passed away: Ah, then it would be my body lying in the coffin; lying there in the dark, waiting to be carried out. It would be my friends and family sitting with glum faces along the pews and someone recounting the highlights

of my life. It would be they who would be wondering how life would be without me; both the good points and the bad. My departure would create a large absence in their lives and in the lives of all the people I was associated with: friends, fellow students, fellow hobbyists, those I have met in the street. . . .

My dying would certainly leave a big hole in their lives; a hole that will take time to accommodate; a hole much like the one Aunty Sue's departure is leaving for us. This is what my own death would be like.

Leo had returned to imagining his own death using images of what he thinks would happen for himself, but this time he had slanted it differently by placing his death in the center of his own social world. In this way my-death was being seen as not only a transition in consciousness but also a transition from his community here on earth and into that community of abiding observers he imagined after death.

The End of Everything

So far, we have seen the way looking at my-death through the lens of other-death throws up several possibilities, including maneuvers where my consciousness is transposed into the consciousness of someone who is dying, the idea of an afterlife where me-as-dead persists in some form, and the idea of a community of abiding observers that I join with when I die. In this way, Leo's responsiveness to the death of his aunt can be seen as involving a triple maneuver. First, he had projected his aunt's soul out of her body and into a higher dimension. His second move was to visualize her entering a preexisting realm, some form of observation platform shared with others who have passed away. His third move was to project his own existence into that same realm. In this way, he was interpreting his own mortality through the lens of what he thinks other-death might be like and, accordingly, to frame his death as a transition into an ever-abiding realm.

However, as stated in opening to this book, my-death, as encountered in its raw essence, is very different from other-death.[13] Other-death, as applied to oneself, draws on the image of the self being projected outside itself thereby enabling us to talk about death as a parting, a leaving, a transition, a going somewhere else. Encounters with my-death, in its true sense, confront us with no such simple way to think or talk about death. It is death stripped of transcendent images or mental maneuvers. What is at stake is not the absence of someone in the world, but the status of the world's existence in itself.[14] My-death poses the unacceptable and unthinkable prospect of not only the final annihilation of myself but also the annihilation of the world and existence as a whole.[15]

Auntie Sue's coffin was carried from the hearse, then laid across the top of the open grave and readied for lowering. Leo noticed how brightly the varnished wood and the metal handles shone in the sunlight. The minister continued where he had left off in the church. In a well-practiced and lilting manner, he talked about God, the consolations of faith, and Aunty Sue's transition into heaven.

After he finished, Leo walked over and stood by the grave, picked up a straw basket and began handing out large camellia petals to the queue of mourners. They each took turns at throwing the petals down onto the coffin. After paying their respects, the circle slowly dispersed and figures could be seen walking back towards their cars. Leo remained standing by the grave looking down on the petal-strewn coffin.

At this moment Leo was struck by the extraordinary and momentous nature of what it meant to be burying Aunty Sue. "We are all here to place her in the ground," he declared to himself. It was an obvious statement, but its full implications were only just dawning on him. "All these people are placing someone they love in the ground; someone who they had shortly before been talking to, doing things with, laughing with, living with. . . . Now they leave her all alone in this dark, shitty hole in the ground."

He looked up to see people still filtering toward their cars. He was now standing by himself next to grave. His mind was calling out, "What are you doing? Hey, you can't just leave her here and walk away! This is Aunty Sue; this is the woman we love and care about." He stared down at the coffin. "We cannot leave this woman lying alone in this cold, cold earth. Surely she can't be left here alone. Surely we can't discard her so easily; casting her off like an old coat. Surely people can't walk away so lightly. This definitely can't be right."

He felt confused. Feelings were erupting and cascading inside his soul. But it wasn't all about Aunty Sue. The scene was telling him something basic about himself. Something he couldn't put into words; something scary, powerful, mysterious, and real.

Leo was connecting with the confusing brutality of someone else's death, but, in the midst of this was something more. He was struggling to put it into words. All he found he could do was wince, aghast at the ruthlessness of the burial; its definiteness, its finality. He could see the enormity of what it meant to abandon someone's body in the ground, to cast it off as something that no longer functioned, but he also sensed that what had happened was signaling something deeper, something more fundamental, something inexpressible about his own mortality. It seemed almost as though his previous other-death positionings—the transposed observer and abiding observers—were no longer viable. They could be seen, in a way, as covering up or distracting from the reality of personal mortality; a reality that challenged existence as a whole; a reality that intimated at the annihilation of the self, the end of consciousness and the world in its entirety.

When faced, as Leo was, with my-death as the end of consciousness, we realize, startlingly, that it entails no longer being present to observe what is going on. The self, as normally understood, ceases to be part of the world; it ceases in its capacity to receive information through the senses, to interact with objects, and for the brain to process all incoming information; indeed, the whole of consciousness will cease to function. My consciousness will no longer be there to participate in experiencing the world.

Mandy turned around and saw her son still standing by himself looking forlornly into the grave. She walked slowly back and stood behind him. Leo noticed her shadow and quickly turned into her embrace.

"Mom, it's not right; it's not right to leave Aunty Sue alone in the ground, is it?" He began to walk away from the grave with his head pressing against Mandy's shoulder.

"It's okay; you don't have to say anything."

As they walked a sudden shower of rain fell and they hurried arm-in-arm for shelter under a tree.

Leo stared out at the rain lashing the grave stones and a cold shiver ran down his spine. "I realize, now, that it's me and me alone that will experience my death." He allowed the brutality of this thought to seep into the innards of his mind. "I cannot really share this with anyone else."

"You don't have to think that way."

He turned around to face Mandy. "No matter what I do, whether I live long or short, have a happy or a miserable life, do good things or only care about myself; no matter what I do, in the end I still face this lonely reality. And nobody else can do it for me or be there with me."

"Hmm, Leo. Yes. It's like that," said Mandy. She scanned across the cemetery. The rain had stopped falling. "C'mon, let's get back to the car before another shower."

Here Leo acknowledged how the real action for him by the graveside was more about himself than his aunt. The paraphernalia of burials—the corpse, the coffin, the grave, the blessings, and the earth—had for him acted collectively to mark the finality of my-death, and it was this that he was accessing and having difficulty expressing. In this awakening he felt the full force of his mortality, something with which he alone had a relationship and which he could not share with anyone else.

Notes

1. Peter Koestenbaum, *The Vitality of Death: Essays in Existential Psychology and Philosophy* (Westport: Greenwood, 1971) pp. 5–6 (authors emphasis removed. The distinction is also discussed by Sami Pihlström in *Death and Finitude* (Lanham: Lexington Books, 2016).
2. Another key writer on death, Jacques Derrida, in his book on the phenomenology of Husserl, *Voice and Phenomenon: Introduction to the Problem of the Sign in Husserl's Phenomenology* (Northwestern University Press, 2011), also distinguishes between "my-death" and what he refers to as "general death."
3. The importance of bereavements in developing an existential awareness regarding my-death is discussed in I. D. Yalom and M. A. Lieberman, "Bereavement and heightened existential awareness," *Psychiatry* (54:4, 334–35, 1991). G. Nouel, "Construction of meaning in the face of mortality," in A. Tomer et al., eds., *Existential and Spiritual Issues in Death Attitudes* (Mahwah: Laurence Erlbaum, 2013) looked at the existential dynamics of the loss of a child for four grieving mothers and discussed their shifting positions with regards to my-death.
4. Evan Thompson in "Empathy and consciousness," *Journal of Consciousness Studies* (8:6–7, 1–32, 2001) pointed out how the study of empathy is critical to forming understandings of the dynamic interrelations between self and other.
5. Much of the research on the effects of exposure to death has occurred with health professionals, particularly doctors and nurses. For example, see K. Howells et al., "Fear of death and dying in medical students," *Medical Education* (20:6, 502–6, 1986), where medical students were surveyed to find that they thought more about death following their exposures to people dying. Also see S. Sinclair, "Impact of death and dying on the personal lives and practices of palliative and hospice care professionals," *Canadian*

Medical Association Journal (183:2, 18–7, 2011), where palliative care professionals were interviewed to find that their exposure to death was linked to shifts in personal perspectives regarding not only my-death but also their approach to life as a whole.

6. P. Boston, A. Bruce, and R. Schreiber in "Existential suffering in the palliative care settings," *Journal of Pain and Symptom Management* (41:3 604–18, 2011) reviewed 64 studies on the existential suffering and anguish experienced by people in palliative care settings.

7. For example, J. Österlind et al. in, "A discourse of silence: Professional carers reasoning about death and dying in nursing homes," *Ageing and Society* (31:4, 529–44, 2011) used focus groups to interview nursing home caregivers in Sweden about their responses to the deaths of those they cared for. They found caregivers oscillated between silence and confrontation.

8. Two interesting studies explored the extent to which soldiers' exposure to threats of dying interacted with psychological processes and religious affiliations: V. Florian and M. Mikulincer, "The impact of death-risk experiences and religiosity on the fear of personal death," *Omega: Journal of Death and Dying* (26:2, 101–11, 1993) and C. van den Berg and J. Soeters, "Self-perceptions of soldiers under threat," *Military Psychology* (21:sup2, S16–30, 2009).

9. Philip C. Almond, *Afterlife: A History of Life After Death* (London: I. B. Tauris, 2016).

10. This is covered in the collection by Y. Nagasawa and B. Matheson (eds.), *The Palgrave Handbook of the Afterlife* (London: Palgrave Macmillan, 2017), and provides an overview of various philosophical and religious interpretations regarding life after death.

11. See J. Edward Wright, *The Early History of Heaven* (New York: Oxford University Press, 2002).

12. The profound significance of heaven for Christianity is described in detail by Jeffrey Burton Russell, *A History of Heaven: The Singing Silence* (Princeton, NJ: Princeton University Press, 1998).

13. The distinction between my-death and other-death aligns with Koestenbaum's analysis in *The Vitality of Death* and draws on Martin Heidegger's concept of Being-unto-death developed in *Being and Time* (Oxford: Basil Blackwell, 1973, 1927).

14. M. Mikulincer and V. Florian in "The complex mulifaceted nature of the fear of personal death," in A. Tomer et al., eds. *Existential and Spiritual Issues in Death Attitudes* (Mahwah: Laurence Erlbaum, 2013) broke fear of my-death into three "dimensions," which they saw as "the intrapersonal, interpersonal, and transpersonal meanings that people can attach to their own death" (p. 42).

15. The unthinkable nature of my own death is discussed more fully by Francoise Dastur in *Death: An Essay in Finitude* (London: Athlone, 1996) and by Zygmunt Bauman in *Mortality, Immortality and Other Life Strategies* (Stanford, CA: Stanford University Press, 1992).

3

Limits of Intelligibility

So, looking at myself from the outside, when I die, my brain will stop working, my senses will cease to operate, I will no longer have any voluntary control of my muscles, and my body will lie limp and lifeless. This is undeniably what will happen.

Looking at this from the inside is more complicated. If my brain and my body cease to function, then it makes sense to consider my emotions, my consciousness, and all those aspects that make up my subjective world as ceasing to operate as well. My consciousness surely relies on input from my senses plus the processing power of my brain so without them it is hard to think of how consciousness might persist. I might reassure myself that my consciousness will continue in some form in another realm, but I can't be sure. It makes more sense to say that when all the conditions for consciousness are no longer present, then my consciousness will no longer be able to function.

But this is terrible thought; a horrifying realization with ghastly consequences. My consciousness is always present whenever I look out at anything in the world. I never experience anything around me without being conscious. When I am unconscious, such as when I am asleep or knocked out, I assume the world continues under its own steam, but this is an assumption which I can never fully trust; well, actually, at the time I'm not really awake to appraise it anyway. What I can be surer about is that the world and my consciousness are always paired; they are always together, with each interacting with the other, each enabling the other, each participating together in allowing what happens to take place.

What this throws up is the possibility that, without my mind the world and all that it contains—objects, animals, people, loved ones—will cease to exist. In other words, from the standpoint of my consciousness, when I die the conditions that enable the existence of both my consciousness and the world around me will, most likely, no longer be present. In this way, the prospect of my own death highlights, as mentioned in the previous chapter, the possibility of the end of everything.[1]

Total Annihilation

Let's take a closer look at what the end of everything might entail. If we embrace the idea that the world's continuation is dependent on my continuing consciousness, where does that lead? In one of his autobiographical works, the Russian writer Leo Tolstoy described his ongoing struggle with the prospect of annihilation as follows:

> *Then these moments of perplexity began to recur oftener and oftener, and always in the same form. They were always expressed by the questions: What is it for?*
>
> *What does it lead to? . . . My life came to a standstill . . . I could not even wish to know the truth, for I guessed of what it consisted. The truth was that life is meaningless. I had as it were lived, lived, and walked, walked, till I had come to a precipice and saw clearly that there was nothing ahead of me but destruction. It was impossible to stop, impossible to go back, and impossible to close my eyes or avoid seeing that there was nothing ahead but suffering and real death—complete annihilation.*[2]

My-death is embedded deep within my bounded consciousness; it sits there menacingly, ready to detonate at any point, ready in one destructive explosion to turn all I am, know, and love into dust and then into nothingness.

Leo sauntered out the front door, sat down in a chair on the veranda, and gazed out over the street. It was a warm day, and a slight breeze was keeping the veranda pleasantly cool.

It was more than six months since his dramatic realization at Aunty Sue's graveside of the enormity of his own mortality. It had shocked him then, and he was still pondering over its implications. Initially he had found himself thinking about it every day, sometimes late into the night, but over the past two weeks he had become more philosophical and less shocked by its implications.

He glanced up the street and noticed Stan approaching from the main road, pulling his grocery cart behind him. He looked hot and stopped occasionally to catch his breath and wipe his forehead.

"Come over here, Stan; take a break, it's nice and cool."

Stan looked up and smiled then wheeled his cart through the gate and left it on the pathway. He stepped up onto the veranda and sat down on the chair next to Leo. "Thanks, it's so hot out there today."

They sat quietly for a few moments while Stan recovered his breath, then he asked, "So, Leo, have you been thinking more about what happened to you at the funeral?"

"Hmm. Yes, a bit. I keep thinking about how everything will end when I die." He smiled incongruously. "You see, what I can't get my head around is that if everything depends on my mind, then, when I die my mind will cease to operate, so then everything else will cease to operate as well."

"You can't be sure about that. It's an assumption."

"No, I can't be sure, but I am sure that things only happen when I'm conscious. So if I'm permanently unconscious it seems fairly likely that, for me at least, the world would cease to be there."

"I don't get it," muttered Stan, a little annoyed. "Why does everything have to grind to a halt when your life ends? The whole of creation doesn't revolve around you."

"No, no, don't get me wrong; not *me* in particular but *me* in the general sense: your-*me* and my-*me*. The same thing would happen to you when you die, but that's your business, not mine."

"Okay, but I have no trouble thinking of things carrying on after I die. It was all there before I was born and it will carry on well after I'm gone."

"Ah, okay, but try thinking of it this way. Can you think of anything that isn't experienced? Do you know anything that hasn't come to you via your experience?"

Stan paused to collect his thoughts, "I guess not." He looked out across the houses. "But what I experience is derived from what's around me. I derive what I experience from what's going on outside. It carries on as it does whether I experience it or not."

"Hah, who's making assumptions now? You can't say it carries on if you're not there to observe it. All you really know is it's there when you experience it, but you have no idea of what's happening when you're not there. And the same goes for death. When you die, you stop experiencing things; you have no access to what lies beyond, so it makes more sense to think of it all as finishing."

Stan shook his head and leaned back in his seat. "Oh, Leo, it's too hard thinking about this stuff in this heat."

Leo's questions about my-death have propelled their discussion into the classic tension in philosophy between realists and idealists. Realists claim the world exists independently of the mind, and idealists view the world and the mind as constantly interacting.[3] Realism draws a solid line between the world as an independent reality and the mind as something that uses perceptions to interpret what is going on. Idealism argues that this line is blurred and that the mind is always actively engaging in constructing what we see as real. Realism is, arguably, the default position because its assumptions are embedded in the way we live our daily lives; we tend to treat the world around as an independently continuing entity. However, when we think more deeply about the nature of reality, about what Alfred North Whitehead referred to as "really real" reality,[4] confidence about the solid and continuous character of the world becomes less clear and the range of ways in which consciousness plays a necessary and constitutive role in what is seen as real becomes more obvious. Various forms of idealism have emerged throughout the history of ideas. In European traditions, idealism has been championed by key thinkers such as Plato, G. W. F. Hegel, and Bishop George Berkeley[5]; in Chinese traditions by Chuang Tsu, Cheng Hao, and Wang Yangming[6]; and in Indian traditions by the ancient *Upanishads* themselves and by thinkers such as Sri Aurobindo and Sarvepalli Radhakrishnan.[7] In more recent times the tenets of idealism are recognizable in the various forms of constructionism with wide applications in sociology, anthropology, social psychology, and in some forms of qualitative research.[8]

What follows from applying an idealist perspective to the nature of my-death is a breakdown in the conditions of reality. When I die, when my consciousness ceases to function, the collaborative partnership between the mind and the world will be severed, which means the way reality is understood will begin to unravel. If the mind is no longer present, its active involvement in constructing the world in which we live can no longer take place. In this way the set of conditions under which what is real takes place collapses into itself and implodes into a nothingness, a total annihilation.

Brenda strolled through the front door to join Leo and Stan on the porch. She sat on the top step in the shade. "Ah, that breeze is really cooling things down."

"Hi, Brenda," greeted Stan, "come and join our debate. Leo here has been arguing that when we die, our consciousness ceases to function, so because our experience of the world is dependent on consciousness, then my individual death entails death of the world as a whole."

"Yes, but more than that," clarified Leo. "Death is final. Nothing exists beyond my dying: no consciousness, no world, no nothing. When my consciousness is annihilated then everything is annihilated."

"Hmm," pondered Brenda. "This is a strong position." She stared out across the street at a boy passing on a red bicycle. "I can see how you might think that way . . . but how can you be sure everything finishes?"

"That's exactly what I asked," interrupted Stan.

"I don't. . . . " replied Leo tentatively. "Look, I don't really want to see it that way, but it's just obviously what happens. It was hard at first, but now it makes total sense. Death is final. Nothing comes after it. There is no 'beyond death' for me or for the world around. When I die, everything finishes."

"Yeah, I've heard what you're saying," said Brenda taking in a deep breath. "But have you thought through what follows on from this? I mean, doesn't it make you wonder about the point of it all? We're born into this world, and, throughout our lives, we strive and strive: we strive to be good by helping others, we strive for success in our jobs, we strive to achieve things like having children and building homes and learning as much as we can, we strive to be good, caring, community-minded people; but it all ends up as zilch. So what's the point of all this striving when the moment we die it all turns into nothingness?"

"I agree," said Stan, "what would be the point? None of us would bother with anything if annihilation is all we can look forward to."

"Okay, okay, I take your point," responded Leo defensively. "Looking at it from above, it would all seem a bit pointless, and, of course, we need some sense of purpose to carry on. But when you get right down inside your consciousness, you can then see how central it is to all that's going on." He glanced at both his listeners to see they were following. "It's a core part of everything that happens to you. . . . So if you conclude that your consciousness stops functioning when you die, then that leads naturally to concluding that everything would be affected."

Speaking from a common-sense point of view, Stan and Brenda argued that the idea of my-death as annihilation lacks any credibility because it would rob everyday life of any meaning or purpose. Leo was inviting them to step beyond an everyday life perspective and to take on board some of the more constitutive ingredients that enable individual consciousness and individual existence to take place. This marks the beginning of an approach to my-death which, for him, will find more organized and confident expression in Chapter 6. In the meantime, despite the incredulity of his listeners, it is worth noting that Leo's idea of my-death as nothingness has been shared by many thinkers, particularly thinkers with idealist tendencies, such as Ludwig Feuerbach and Arthur Schopenhauer, and more recently Jay Rosenberg and Jean-Paul Sartre.[9]

Not Even Annihilation

According to Leo, intimations of my-death point toward the ultimate breakdown of the interdependence between consciousness and the world of things that exist and that this breakdown can be thought of as nothingness or annihilation. But is this the only way that this breakdown could be interpreted? There might be other ways of approaching it.

It was mid-week, and Brenda began a well-earned day off by hanging her week's washing out on the line. She relished this time to herself and was enjoying the warmth of the early morning sun. She looked back toward the house and noticed Stan walking along the side of the house.

"Hi, Brenda," greeted Stan. "I'm just returning this garden fork I borrowed the other day."

Brenda stopped pegging out her clothes and beckoned him to the chairs in the yard. "Stan, have a seat for a moment. I've something I'd like to talk over."

They settled into the chairs, which had been pleasantly warmed by the sun. Brenda opened the discussion, "You know how Leo's been talking to us about death?" Stan nodded. "Well, I've had real difficulties knowing how to respond; what to say, particularly around his claims of death as a final end." She glanced across at Stan. "What do you make of what he's saying?"

"I'm struck by how adamant he is about finality, particularly his view that when we . . . excuse me, I mean, when I die, what will follow is the end of everything; it will be a final nothingness."

"That's it," said Brenda leaning forward. "I also have trouble with this view. To me it seems rather glib, almost too simple; like he's kind of relishing taking such an absolute position." She sat back and allowed the sun to soak over her face. "But I really struggle to challenge him on it."

"Let's see if together we might understand it a little better," Stan suggested hesitantly, a little unsure where the conversation might lead. "He's talking about the end of his consciousness as a final nothingness, as eternal oblivion, and he bases that on everything being dependent on me—my 'me,' not yours—being present as a conscious experiencer." Stan paused briefly to consider what he'd just said. "I can see what he's wanting to say, but I think he's jumped a bit ahead of himself."

"Yeah, but how? I can appreciate the finality of death, but then he jumps into his talk of annihilation. I don't see how finality necessarily leads to annihilation."

"Hmm, I know . . . I know where he's taken things a bit far," said Stan leaning forward in his chair. "See, we only know about annihilation by observing things that get annihilated. One moment something is there, the next moment it's disappeared; yesterday my living room was crawling with ants, then I sprayed it and all the ants were annihilated; until 1220, a hundred thousand people lived in Samarkand, then Genghis Khan annihilated the whole population. Things are there, ants and people, then they go, but their going takes place against the backdrop of where they existed. The room in which the ants used to crawl around is still there; the place where the people of Samarkand used to live is still there; annihilation only makes sense against a backdrop upon which an absence can be registered."

"So you're saying that for us to think annihilation we need to see it as a disappearance occurring against some form of continuing background. Something needs to continue against which the idea of annihilation makes sense. It's kind of like the term defeats itself." She looked down at her watch. "Oh, is that the time? I have to get going." She stood up and smiled down at Stan. "You stay here as long as you like."

Here, Stan was beginning to clarify how issues of my-death might have less to do with the nature of existence and more to do with the nature of language. Leo's talk of my-death as annihilation drew on a word we normally use within the context of something that has disappeared. But discontinuation only makes sense in front of a backdrop of ongoing continuation; applying the concept of annihilation to the end of consciousness, the end of the world, and the end of all existence extends its use well beyond where it is capable of operating. In a way, saying that nothingness occurs at the end of my life could also be understood as saying that nothing can be said about the end of my life, and speaking this way is more akin to the language of poetry where possibilities are intimated or hinted at rather than boldly asserted.

The challenges for language in this arena become more apparent when one system of speaking comes up against and clashes with an entirely different system of speaking.

Leo took a break from his study and joined Mandy in the living room. She was sitting with her legs curled up on the couch browsing through a magazine. He sat in the armchair opposite her.

"Mom, what do you think happens when you die?"

"Well," she replied continuing to browse, "life just carries on. You have to carry on, don't you?"

"No, I mean, when you die, what happens to you?"

"Well, I dunno," said Mandy pausing her browsing and looking slightly annoyed at the interruption. "I guess, if you've lived a good life you go to heaven and from there you can watch the world continue on in your absence."

"Aww, Mom, you don't really think that happens? That's what you said when I was a child. But now, well, heaven and hell, and angels and all that; it's just not credible. What I reckon is that when you die, there's nothing further."

"Look, Leo," she said putting down her magazine, "you're still young and have lots to learn. You're not really ready to take on such confusing topics. It'll just muck your head around."

"Okay, okay," he said with playful energy. "Let's just look a little closer at what you're claiming. Show me the proof that you're gonna live on after you die. Is there any solid evidence for there being a heaven or some other form of afterlife?"

Mandy replied slowly and reluctantly, wondering how she might close down such an uncomfortable conversation. "These things are hard to prove because they belong to another realm; the realm of the soul."

"Same question. Is there any evidence that this other realm exists?"

"Oh, Leo, I don't know. I'm sure there is some evidence. But do you really need evidence? We're obviously here for a reason." Her tone was becoming increasingly strident. "Does having evidence really matter?"

"Well, yes, it does actually because . . . because if you can't give me any good reason for thinking otherwise, I'm going to continue seeing death as the end of everything."

"Leo, stop it, stop it right now," she stated loudly, her face quivering with emotion. "Believe me, this is not a topic you should be thinking about. And, as your mother, I'm pleading with you—no I'm demanding—that you stop immediately any further thoughts or talk about this topic."

"Ah, it's pointless talking about this with you." With that he strode resolutely out of the living room, slamming the door behind him.

Leo has stumbled across another area of strong debate: How similar or how different should we approach the languages of science and religion? Both forms of speaking are making claims on the nature of reality. The language of science establishes its legitimacy by means of clear definition, precise measurement, and repeated observation. The language of religion establishes its legitimacy more by means of universal concepts, revealed wisdom, and divine intimations. Some theorists have argued that religious language is able to venture into territories that science is unable to go, and it achieves this by means of a system of metaphorical concepts.[10] Others have argued, more controversially, that the languages of science and religion are not so different because the key concepts of science—such as energy and force—rely on a similar use of metaphors and, when more closely examined, reveal similar levels of universality and vagueness.[11] Either way, it highlights the diversity of options we have available for thinking and talking about ultimate reality.

Beyond Thinking

What the argument between Mandy and Leo has thrown up is the challenge of reaching some form of consensus as to what it means to die. Different ways of speaking come up with alternative ideas, and, unfortunately, these ideas tend to contradict each other, leaving little room for accommodation. Whether life continues on in some form after dying or whether it ends in total oblivion, the disagreement not only relates to the lack of access to information about what will happen but is also linked to the language systems out of which these ideas have emerged. Perhaps by shifting our focus from the nature of my-death to looking at it as a problem associated with the bounds of thought and bounds of language, we might find some basis for reaching a consensus.

"Hellooo, anyone home?" called out Leo as he walked through Stan's kitchen heading toward his living room.

Stan strolled out of his bedroom rubbing his eyes. "Leo, good to see you. Go and sit down in the living room, I've got something to show you." From a trunk behind his couch he pulled out a tatty photo album and rummaged through its leaves. "You know how I used to be in the Marines and managed to serve three tours in Vietnam?"

"I know about your time in. . . . "

"There, that's the photo. Look here; look at this." He turned the album around so Leo could lean forward and examine the faded photo. "This is the remains of a village I visited after it was strafed by jets. See, everything in it, every house, every fence, every structure was annihilated by the bombs. All you have is the village's shattered remains."

"Ah, I get it. I know what you're getting at. . . . You're trying to make a point about what happens when things get annihilated."

"Yes, don't you see? We can only talk about annihilation by referencing what was there and then by referencing what remains. The village was there in the terrain, now there is just the terrain. But I can't talk of annihilation as a total nothingness. It takes the word too far away from how we use it. I think what you are doing is talking about annihilation as though it can stand there in its own right." He paused to study Leo's perplexed expression. "But you can only do that by contrasting it with something that remains, something that continues."

"Okay, I see your point," acknowledged Leo as he sank back with a sigh into the armchair. "Annihilation implies some form of continuation. But it's the best word I can think of to capture what I'm getting at. Are you saying my ideas on finality aren't any good?"

"No, I think your ideas on death are just as good as mine. You say everything finishes at death, and I have a sense that the world carries on after it. But neither of us can be sure . . . and neither of us is confident about how to say what we mean."

"Hmm, but we both can't be right . . . or can we?"

"I don't think it's a matter of whose right or wrong," said Stan. "I think we both want to say something about what happens when we die, but neither of us can really say it. That's the problem. Every word we choose doesn't quite deliver what we want. For you it's 'nothingness,' 'final end,' 'annihilation'; creation next to its destruction, ongoing life next to a final end, and . . . ah, ah . . . somethingness next to nothingness and so on. But none of these does justice to what you mean by death's finality. For me it's 'continuation,' 'transcendence,' and 'diffusion'; I have this vague sense that the world and my soul, or my spirit, or some sort of cosmic presence, continues on."

"I suppose, in a way, by talking of annihilation and nothingness, I'm pointing to death as though it's a bit like a black hole; an unobservable particularity that we have no way of knowing anything about. Hah, I guess I'm agreeing with you; death is a location of total mystery."

"If anything, when it comes to our differing philosophical positions, I'd prefer to say we're both right. I think what you and I are both trying to tell each other, in different ways, is that when it comes to my own death what happens is totally unknowable."

"I think you mean more that it is fundamentally unthinkable."

"Yes, that's what I think we are agreeing on. When I turn and stare straight at my own death, what I somehow sense is that there is no direct or legitimate way for me to attempt to describe it; it's then I realize it's completely unthinkable . . . unknowable . . . and unintelligible."

In the face of neither Leo nor Stan being willing to accept the other's position, they were willing to consider a compromise in which both their conceptualizations (annihilation vs. continuation) are understood as partial attempts to address the fundamental unthinkability and unspeakability of my-death. They recognized the inherent weakness in both their positions. It is neither confidently global annihilation nor confidently a continuing afterlife; both are acceptable and neither are acceptable. In this ambiguous and uncertain space resides the unintelligibility of my-death; it just cannot be thought, described, or interpreted. My-death hangs there as a threat, somehow suspended between afterlife and annihilation. An unthinkable space of high anxiety.

As will be explored more closely in Chapter 5, the unintelligibility of my-death creates a barrier to finding a way of establishing a secure and definitive understanding of my-death. It prevents my-death from coalescing into an object of experience that has sufficient conceptual integrity for the mind to engage and talk about. It drives us toward more indirect and figurative ways of thinking and speaking.

"Hi, Stan," said Brenda as she stood at his front door on his porch. "I thought I'd take up your offer of a coffee and biscuits."

"Come on through." He led her into his small, tightly arranged kitchen with a small wooden table pushed up against the wall. He signaled for her to sit at the table, and he busied himself with preparing the coffee. "In the future it might be better to come through the kitchen door; there's a much quicker route through that gap in the fence."

"Okay, I'll do that." She smiled as she recognized this as an invitation for further visits. She sat down at the table on the chair against the wall. "How's it all going?"

"Well, I'm having regular visits and discussions with Leo. Mostly we talk about death. It's the only thing he seems willing to talk about since Sue's funeral."

"He's certainly stirred things up," commented Brenda. "I've struggled to answer his many questions."

"At first I thought it was just a reaction, so I didn't pay much attention. But, if anything, his interest has got more intense. I find it a bit unnerving."

"What, because of what he's saying?"

"Well, it's just that his questions are forcing me to think about where I stand." Stan placed the coffee mugs and a plate of cookies on the table and sat down. "And I just don't know what to think. It's a solid brick wall I can't think beyond. In my head, I think he's right: my death will be the end of everything. In my heart, I don't think he's right but I'm not sure why."

"Me, too. I have no trouble talking about other people's death. I do that every day as part of my job. But his focus on his and our own deaths is a bit disconcerting. Maybe . . . maybe because I don't know what to say."

"Yes, last time I talked to Leo we ended up agreeing that, as far as my own death is concerned, its nature is fundamentally unthinkable. We might try to apply concepts like nothingness or afterlife, but these are approximations; they're vaguely formed metaphors or working hypotheses. . . . Whatever they are, they have little chance of forming into clearer concepts."

"Hmm, maybe that's why people avoid thinking about death. Perhaps it's because we can't think about it that we avoid it."

"That's true," agreed Stan. "The scariest things in my life are things that are vague, uncertain, and difficult to describe: I fear being disabled, I fear the big spider that might be lurking in the corner, I fear people disapproving of me, I fear how others might judge my achievements. . . . Like my own death, I don't want to think about these things; I push to them into a little box at back of my mind and try hard to never let them escape that confinement."

Stan was suggesting that the unthinkable and unspeakable nature of my-death in some way links up with the way we often struggle with or at least try to avoid thinking about it. It is almost as though our embrace of life varies to the extent that we turn our backs on death.

Added to this are other layers that contribute to what makes it scary to think about my-death.[12] My-death connects in various ways to how we experience the death of other people. The occasional thoughts of the death of a parent, a partner, or a child can, at unexpected moments, fill us with dread. This might relate to fears of having to watch loved ones die, fears of final separation, and fears of continuing on in a life without them. As with my-death, the fear is amplified by not knowing when this might occur. Another layer of scariness relates to our ability to project ourselves into the death of others: it is frightening to think of the pain and suffering of close family members following one's own death, it is alarming to think of our bodies entering a crematorium furnace or being lowered into a grave, and it is perplexing to think of the world continuing on without us once our death registers us as an absence. Another layer of scariness concerns our fears of the dying process itself: our fear of potential pain, of having to observe the distress of loved ones, and of not being able to cope with the trauma of leaving. All aspects associated with these three additional layers of scariness connect in a general way with what makes death, in all its various forms, a fearsome topic and one that should be avoided.

However, if we were to imagine stripping away these three additional layers of fear and to look at my-death just on its own, the uncertainties that surround it and its essential mysteriousness can be seen as fear-promoting in their own right. This was what Stan and Brenda were concluding. The unthinkable and unspeakable nature of my-death forces us to walk repeatedly down a conceptual dead-end—a dead-end which discourages any further attempts to think along the same track. Even if we were to consider it important to form some sort of relationship to my-death, there is no identifiable object to connect with, there is nothing to cling on to; it stands there as a conceptual black-hole, an emptiness which we can only approach with insecurity and foreboding.

This is the primary challenge undertaken in this book. My-death is too important a topic to neglect and continually skirt around. But how might we enter into some form of relationship with my-death when it appears so impenetrably unspeakable? What frames of reference could we use to pursue a lifelong engagement with my-death? These are the questions around which the remaining chapters of this book will orbit. But, before exploring these possibilities, the next chapter will look more specifically at what it means to be afraid of my-death.

Notes

1. Christopher Belshaw, in *Annihilation: The Sense and Significance of Death* (Stockfield: Acumen, 2009), looks at the dynamics of annihilation at death in a more biological fashion. Drawing on how we speak of death, he highlights how the "irreversible breakdown of the organism" (p. 16) holds most our conceptions of death together.
2. Leo Tolstoy, *A Confession: The Gospel in Brief, and What I Believe* (Oxford University Press, 1940), pp. 15, 17–18.
3. In the social sciences, idealism is often seen as aligned to "constructionism," where the world is viewed as generated through constructs or internal models.
4. Alfred North Whitehead, *Process and Reality* (New York: Free Press, 1978) p. 289.
5. An interesting collection of German traditions in idealism is provided in R. C. Solomon and K. M. Higgins, *The Age of German Idealism* (London: Routledge, 2003).
6. The key ingredients of Chinese idealism are beautifully captured by Chang Chung-Yuan in *Creativity and Taoism: A Study of Chinese Philosophy, Art and Poetry* (London: Wildwood House, 1963).
7. An overview of Indian idealist philosophy is provided by Surendranath Dasgupta, *Indian Idealism* (Cambridge: Cambridge University Press, 1933).
8. In an early and influential book on constructionism, P. Berger and T. Luckmann, *The Social Construction of Reality* (London: Penguin Books), lay out the central ideas for constructivism in the social sciences.
9. Bernard Schumacher in *Death and Mortality in Contemporary Philosophy* (Cambridge: Cambridge University Press, 2010) covers these and other philosophers regarding their position on my-death as nothingness. This is also developed by Jay Rosenberg in *Thinking Clearly About Death* (Indianapolis: Hackett Publishing, 1998). Jean-Paul Sartre developed his ideas on death in several books, particularly in *Being and Nothingness* (New York: Washington Square Press, 1992).
10. Examples of studies on the rhetorical elements in religious language include Janet Soskice, *Metaphor and Religious Language* (Oxford: Clarendon Press, 1985), and David Tacey, *Religion as Metaphor: Beyond Literal Belief* (Abingdon Oxon: Routledge, 2017).
11. The similarities between the languages of science and religion are examined by E. R. MacCormac, "Religious metaphors," *Zygon* (18, 45–65, 1983) and I. G. Barbour, *Religion and Science* (San Francisco: HarperCollins, 2013).
12. Fear of death will be covered in more detail in the following chapter.

4

Aversion and Evasion

To what extent should my-death be viewed as a positive or negative part of life?

On the one hand, my-death plays a vital role in structuring existence and enabling it to have value and meaning: for instance, how can an event in life be seen as having any value if it keeps on repeating itself in an endless sequence? On the other hand, my-death can also be considered as the source of all loss and destruction: it represents the prospect of the ultimate annihilation—annihilation not just of myself but of the whole of creation.

This dilemma has played out along cultural trajectories throughout history, particularly in the form of ambiguously portrayed personifications of death. For example, the ancient Greek god of nonviolent death, Thanatos, was at times depicted as a benign figure accompanying the recently dead into the underworld, but in other contexts he was referred to in more negative ways as having "a heart of iron" and as being "pitiless as bronze."[1] The Valkyrie of Norse mythology were female figures who played the role of determining who would live or die in battle, which led the average Viking to both respect and fear them in equal measure.[2] Similarly, the Angel of Death (mal'ake ha-mavet) of ancient Jewish faith was sometimes sent by God to slay large numbers of enemies, but he was also prone to target the Israelites themselves, thereby qualifying him of both their respect and their fear. This ambivalence shifted in the fourteenth century when the Black Death swept through the cities and towns of Europe taking with it the lives of a third to a half of their inhabitants.[3] Such merciless carnage tipped the balance in favor of death as something to be feared. Death found itself embodied in the formidable image of the Grim Reaper, a skeleton in a black cloak wielding a scythe who harvested people's lives in a wholesale and indiscriminate fashion.[4]

Through the following centuries such negative imagery maintained and, at times, strengthened this general fear of death—at least in European cultures—by linking it to macabre images such as skeletons, skulls, blood, ghosts, ghouls, and gravestones.[5] Consider, for example, the way in which piracy came to be represented by the image of a skull and crossbones. But beneath this generalized uneasiness lurked a more specific fear, a fear that resists description and confounds direct thought: the fear associated both with the possibility and inevitability of my-death. It is this more specific fear and, as discussed in the previous chapter, its unintelligibility which can be seen, arguably, to propel the unsettling energy behind the various general representations of death.

Ernest Becker, in his influential 1973 book *The Denial of Death*, argued that fear of my-death is hardwired into us and, as such, can act as a barrier to our full appreciation of life.[6]

> *The irony of man's condition is that the deepest need is to be free of the anxiety of death and annihilation; but it is life itself which awakens it, and so we must shrink from being fully alive.[7]*

Becker contended that this collective denial, which serves to protect us from the unthinkable horror of my-death, is achieved by means of various "immortality projects," systems of stories and beliefs often derived from religious faiths, which help us maintain a sense of immortality which, in turn, enables us to function through our daily lives.

> *The knowledge of death is reflective and conceptual, and animals are spared it. They live and they disappear with the same thoughtlessness: a few minutes of fear, a few seconds of anguish, and it is over. But to live a whole lifetime with the fate of death haunting one's dreams and even the most sun-filled days— that's something else. . . . I believe that those who speculate that a full apprehension of man's condition would drive him insane are right, quite literally right.[8]*

In other words, immortality belief systems allow us to turn away from the incomprehensible reality of my-death and pursue daily life in ways that avoid being wracked by the anxiety of what will happen to us at the end of our lives.

Other writers have argued that fear of death comes from more cultural and, accordingly, more modifiable origins. For example, James Brain (1979) contended that the topics of both sex and death are two of the last taboos, the last main spaces in which open discussion is not condoned.[9] This is interesting because, since he published his book, the taboos around sex have shifted radically, but open discussion about death, particularly my-death, still remains awkward territory. But that does not imply that conversations about death, given the right circumstances, are incapable of becoming a more common and more comfortable activity. As with sex, talking about death could over time become an acceptable topic. More recently Raymond Lee (2008) has challenged the whole idea of a taboo,[10] and Ruth McManus (2012) has placed death awareness in a global context and has argued that not only do approaches differ between cultures, but also that they are undergoing constant change due to pressures from the "fast evolving practices of globalization" fueled by media, technology, and the internet.[11]

Fear of Death

Now, let's take a closer look at how fear of my-death plays out in modern Western societies. There are many intriguing aspects, not the least of which is a fundamental ambivalence toward my-death and all it represents.

Leo marched through Stan's kitchen into his living room, where he found him bending forward in his armchair squinting at a book under the light from the window.

"What'ya reading?" enquired Leo as he plonked down on the couch and began fiddling with the curtains. He enjoyed the casual freedom of their relationship and Stan's encouragement for him to drop in unannounced whenever he pleased.

"Ah, hi Leo. It's a book that Brenda lent me. It's called *Death* by Shelly Kagan; he's a philosopher from Yale."[12]

"The book sounds cheerful." He stopped fiddling with the curtain, glanced across at Stan and asked, "What's Brenda trying to suggest?"

"No, no. She's not trying to suggest anything . . . certainly not that I should prepare for death. The topic just came out of our conversations about her work. She recommended it because it covers many of the issues we've been discussing. I just said I wouldn't mind reading it, and so she got it for me."

"Okay, so what's it telling you?"

"Well, it's interesting. It's made me think about a lot of things: whether the soul actually exists, whether life continues after death, what it means to die . . . lots of things." Stan sat back in his armchair and stared at the sunlight dancing around the curtain. "But overall, I find the topic difficult and perplexing. Whenever I think about it, my mind ends up spinning off in different directions and not staying on any topic in particular."

"Like it's avoiding something?"

"Hmm, that's right. And then, after a while, I keep coming back to this same disturbing thought." He turned toward at Leo and with a faint smile on his face. "It often seems like . . . like, ah, if death were a person, he would be laughing at each of us; laughing at our efforts to be successful, to be good, to live meaningful lives. No matter what I try to achieve, death and not me is the winner in the end."

"Hah. So what's the point?" exclaimed Leo. "What's the point of trying at all because no matter who you are: no matter how good, how healthy, how rich or how adored; no matter who you are, we all arrive at the same place."

"Yes, it's the ultimate leveler."

Stan was intrigued by the various issues that my-death raised, but he found it equally difficult to stay focused and do justice to this fascination. He wanted to develop his understanding of death, but with each attempt he became flustered and confused and often ended up backing away. His beliefs about death seemed at odds with how he behaved toward it.

For social scientists, the murky territory between beliefs and behavior, particularly those involving ambivalence and active evasion, has been of particular interest. Indeed, American psychology of the 1950s and 1960s witnessed a wide range of research programs aimed at better understanding challenging topics such as sex and sexuality, obedience and conformity, gender bias and racial stereotypes. For example, we might like to think of ourselves as autonomous and independent beings, but studies on obedience have revealed how much of our social behavior can be shaped and influenced by the people around us.[13] Such research drew to a large extent on ways of measuring beliefs and behaviors through the use of standard sets of questions which, after a long period of development, came to be referred to as standardized questionnaires or "scales." Not surprisingly, the beliefs and behaviors associated with death seemed a suitable space to apply these methods, and several standardized questionnaires were developed. Chief among them was the Fear of Death Scale, first published in 1969 by Lora-Jean Collett and David Lester and consisting of a standardized set of thirty-six statements such as "I would avoid death at all costs" and "I am disturbed by the shortness of life." The statements were grouped into four subscales labeled: "death of self," "death of others," "dying of self," and "dying of others."[14]

People endorsed each statement across six options between "strong agreement" and "strong disagreement," and their responses were combined into a score for each subscale.

Early work with Fear of Death Scale focused on whether fear would vary with general personal characteristics such as age, gender, occupation (e.g., being a nurse or a skydiver), and exposure to illness or mental health challenges.[15] Surprisingly, researchers using the scale were, over time, unable to establish any consistent relationships with these characteristics; in other words, being a man or a woman, a nurse or a skydiver, did not appear to affect how afraid a person was of death.[16] Being a person who was more generally prone to anxiety did appear to coincide with being more fearful of death, but this was not surprising nor particularly helpful.[17] However, one curious relationship did emerge: those with religious affiliations seemed to be more likely to fear death.[18] This seemed on the face of it to run counter to Becker's idea that beliefs in immortality common in religious faiths acted as an antidote to the terrifying prospect of my-death. Over the next three decades this odd finding attracted ongoing research interest, and, as death scales improved, the link between religious belief and fear of death emerged as more complicated than first thought. Indeed, contrary to initial findings, some studies found that people with strong religious convictions could be more comfortable about my-death.[19] So faith seems to be associated with greater and lesser fear of death. How can both be right? This was most perplexing.

Brenda arrived home from work to find Leo stretched out on the couch watching an episode of the *Game of Thrones*. She took her coat off, placed her bags down, then went into the kitchen, poured out two glasses of orange juice, and returned to the living room.

"Here, Leo, take a sip of this."

Leo sat up, paused the program, and turned to face Brenda as she handed over the glass then settled into the armchair by the window. "How did it go at work today?"

"Ah, fine," she answered vaguely. "How was your day?"

"Brenda," asked Leo carefully, "Brenda, do people you work with handle their deaths differently?"

"Well that's an interesting question." She placed her glass on a side table and stared up at a small cobweb in the corner of the ceiling. "I guess everything changes when you find out your death's coming sooner rather than later. But, oh, there's all sorts of different responses. Some people are angry at having to leave so soon, some are resigned to their fate, others look forward to what they see as the next phase, some are confused and try as much as possible not to think about it . . . and others are simply terrified."

"Hmm," mused Leo. "I guess you talk with them about what they see happening when they die?"

"Well, yes, some think when they die that's it, it's all over. Others talk of it as a transition to a new life, a life where the soul-minus-body continues on in some ethereal space like heaven. These are usually people with strong religious beliefs."

"I guess it's easier to see yourself continuing on in some way after death."

"Um, it's not always like that. Some people with strong faiths seem more worried . . . even more terrified by death; then others are less worried. . . . I dunno, you can't really predict who's going to find it troubling. I find it all very confusing."

In 1985, Ronald Aday set out to understand these relationships better by asking 123 Israeli Jews to complete the more complex multidimensional scale, the Fear of Personal Death Scale.[20] His results suggested that both fear of death and religious belief seemed to be connecting at a more fundamental level with what he referred to as "basic human concerns."[21] Ann Downey (1984) was heading in a similar direction when she took a closer look at her surveys with middle-aged US men and suggested that the relationship between religiosity and fear of death was "curvilinear."[22] By this she meant that those who believed strongly in either there being or not being an afterlife were less fearful of death than those with weaker beliefs either way. In other words, people who are least likely to fear death are either those with strong nonreligious convictions, such as atheists or agnostics, or those with very strong religious beliefs, such as devout Catholics or Muslims. Wink and Scott (2005) backed up this curvilinear hypothesis when they used data from a Californian longitudinal study to look at how religious belief and fear of death connected for 155 people in late adulthood.[23] More recently, Ellis and Wahab (2013) reviewed eighty-four studies on this topic and, after looking at a number of competing explanations, identified the curvilinear as a promising explanation.[24] Similarly, Jonathan Jong and colleagues (2017) reviewed 100 studies on the topic and looked more closely at the evidence for the curvilinear hypothesis. They concluded:

> *Although our meta-analyses did not provide direct evidence for the curvilinearity hypothesis, and only weak indirect evidence in the form of small negative correlations, a closer examination of the 11 studies that deliberately tested a curvilinear relationship is suggestive.*[25]

So, at this stage, following three decades of research, we can fairly confidently claim that the relationship between fear of death and religious beliefs is complex and that, while evidence for it as a curvilinear relationship has yet to be firmly established, it seems likely that fear of death connects in some way with how certain or uncertain we regard our continuation in some form of afterlife.

Active Evasion

Fear, often seen as primarily a negative emotion, has evolved in us as a way of guiding our behavior to increase our chances of survival. For example, many of our common fears, such as a fear of heights or a fear of poisonous spiders, help guide us away from contexts where danger lurks. However, some of these specific and functional fears can coalesce into more general and less focused fears. For example, a specific fear of poisonous spiders might generalize into a fear of all insects and then spread further to include all situations where insects are likely to be crawling.[26] Such generalized fears can severely constrain where we go and what we do. As a further step, when these generalized fears become shared with other people, when whole groups of people share the same experience, the fear and its associated avoidant behavior can become normalized; they become a shared and commonly understood ways of thinking and behaving.[27] For example, in a classroom, fear of speaking in front of others can reach a point where the whole class ends up viewing evasion as normal, which can leave the teacher floundering for ways to encourage class discussion.

Fear of death can occur in all these various ways. For example, the specific fear of coming into contact with a corpse could have survival value in helping us avoid the transfer of disease and infections. This specific fear can also generalize to a fear of anything associated with death, such as coffins, graves, and mortuaries. When collections of people, perhaps whole societies, accept such generalized fears as normative, avoidance of anything to do with death can turn into a standard practice.

"You look like you've got a lot on your mind?" Mandy enquired as Leo sauntered into the kitchen and sat down at the table opposite her.

Leo gazed pensively at the void outside the window. "Hmm, Mom, I do." He paused. "Mom, what do you think happens to you when you die?"

"Goodness." She looked up and studied her son's expression. "Have you been talking to Brenda?"

"Maybe." He turned and stared across at Mandy. "But really, Mom, what do you think goes on when we die?"

"I dunno. . . ." She shrugged her shoulders and leaned across to the coffee-pot to fill up her mug. "I don't like to think about it. I reckon thinking about it is a bit, a bit . . . well, it's a bit morbid really."

"Morbid?" He looked up. "Ah . . . no . . . I don't understand?"

"I mean that you won't gain much out of thinking about death, other than getting confused or depressed, or both. No, there's not much point in it, thinking about it, I mean. You need to get on with actually living life."

"I don't see it as morbid. I find it fascinating. I don't see why we can't talk about it. We talk about lots of other difficult topics . . . like sex, relationships, and war."

"Well, no point dwelling on something that's so negative you can't do anything about it." This reinforced in her mind concerns that her son was being distracted by issues that could derail his progress in life. "Have you finished that essay?"

"You've changed the topic. Why don't you give me a straight answer?"

Mandy folded the newspaper and placed it on the pile of other papers at the end of the bench. She stood staring at the wall. "Look, I've got other things on my mind. Perhaps we can talk about it another time."

What drives Mandy's reluctance to talk about death and to label such talk as "morbid"? Does her avoidance of the topic have something to do with being reminded of negative and distressing instances of other people's death? Or is it driven by another more fundamental impulse, perhaps by an unwillingness to consider aspects of the reality of her own death?

Fear of death in its various forms—specific, generalized, and normative—provide the impetus and a rationale for actively avoiding thinking and talking about anything to do with death. This can be achieved in a variety of ways. In conversations we might change the topic, as Mandy did when Leo sought her views on my-death. In our thoughts we might distract ourselves onto other topics. In our behavior we might turn away or walk away from situations where things associated with death are likely to crop up. And beneath all these forms of active evasion lies the collective view of my-death as something worthy of avoiding; it helps us to view evasion as a legitimate and permissible activity. This collective view forms the basis for monitoring and judging not only the appropriateness of our own behavior but also the behavior of others.

Brenda backed through the outside door into the kitchen and struggled to pull through two large bags of groceries. "Hi, Mandy; I've bought some provisions." She heaved the bags onto the kitchen bench. "Where's Leo?"

"He has basketball practice tonight. He won't be home 'til after nine."

Brenda walked off to her bedroom to change out of her work clothes then returned to help Mandy with the cooking.

"I've been a little surprised by some of what Leo is coming up with lately." Mandy was staring down at the onions browning in the pan. "He's young and impressionable, you know."

"I'm not sure I follow." Brenda paused from cutting up the chicken breasts and stared across at Mandy. "Are you concerned about something I've been talking to him about?"

"Well, yes, actually, I do have some concerns."

Brenda placed her knife down, turned fully toward Mandy, and crossed her arms. The tension was now palpable, and both knew they were locked on to seeing this through. "Okay, say what you mean."

Mandy continued to look down into the pan. "Look, it's not my business to monitor what you two talk about, but don't you think he's a bit young to handle conversations about death, particularly about his own death?"

"Mandy, I appreciate he's young and death is a tough topic, but it's not me who is bringing it up; he's the one who starts talking about it. Look, he's naturally curious and, I guess, fascinated with what I do for a living." Brenda relaxed her hands onto the benchtop. "Besides which, I reckon it's a good thing that he thinks about such matters."

"Okay, that's it, that's where we differ." She looked up from the pan and stared directly at Brenda. "Personally, I don't think a young man at his age can benefit from a head filled with such negativity. It's gloomy, morbid . . . and unnatural. It could lead him into an unhealthy obsession, perhaps resulting in melancholy or depression . . . or worse."

"I don't think so. I think he's more likely to be troubled by constantly trying to avoid the topic. It's something he and all of us have to come to terms with."

Mandy could feel pressure mounting in her throat. "No, but I. . . ."

Brenda detected her distress and replied, "Okay, okay. Let's just leave it. You're his Mom. I'll try not to talk about it with him in the future. Okay? Leave it like that."

Mandy felt entitled to complain to Brenda about her talking to her son about death because she saw it as normal to avoid such discussions. To her surprise, Brenda challenged her assumption that talking about death was morbid. The challenge was unexpected and unsettling. Brenda recognized this, and, in the interests of household harmony, she backed down.

Strategic Immortality

Common disapproval—or prohibition—of thinking or talking about my-death sets the scene for a range of avoidant behaviors that include euphemistic language, topic diversion, and social disapproval. Such practices not only reduce the likelihood of my-death conversations, but they also open up space for something else. They increase our capacity to pretend, on a day-to-day basis, that we are not going to die, and it is this pretense of personal immortality that forms a protective bubble that frees us from mind-numbing thoughts about my-death.

Brenda had positioned a garden chair in a spot by the fence that captured the last beams of the late afternoon sun. Through slits in the fence, she could just make out Stan's figure shuffling around in his back yard.

"Come over here, Stan; join me in a glass of wine."

"Ah, Brenda, what a good idea. I'll be with you in a shake." He sidled awkwardly through the gap at the end of the fence.

She studied him as he lowered his body carefully into the garden chair next to her. She poured him a glass of wine and placed it next to him on the garden table. "Been busy Stan?"

"Yes, always things to do." He shielded his eyes from the glare. "How was your day?"

"Hmm, the dying business; it's always demanding."

They both sat quietly sipping their wine and allowing the sun's warmth to soak into their joints.

"You know, Brenda, for much of my life I've acted as if I am going to live forever."

Brenda glanced across, a little surprised at this admission. "As you age, Stan, don't you find that gets a little bit harder each year?"

"No, it seems much the same; not something I dwell on much. Don't you do the same?"

"Um, yeah, even though I spend all day with the dying, I still carry on as though dying's never going to happen to me."

"I guess the idea of me dying just doesn't seem to fit in with anything else; like it belongs to some other sphere. Odd, isn't it?"

"Yes, very odd. When I think about it, I know this sense of my life carrying on and on just isn't accurate. Deep inside, I know I will die. My death is a solid and unmistakable condition of me being here." She took another thoughtful sip of her wine. "But, since my early years, while I might think I'm going to die, I don't act or live as if I will. I wake up, eat breakfast, travel to work, go about my business, attend to relationships; all the while assuming that I will continue, that the people around me will continue, and that the world around me will carry on as it always has."

"Yep, that's right. On and on I go, never really thinking about it all finishing." Stan sighed and drained the wine from his glass. "Bit crazy, really. I know I don't have that many years left and yet I still keep pretending it's going to carry on."

"Sometimes thoughts do intrude into my mind; usually an anxious flash: perhaps today I will have a terrible accident, perhaps I will be diagnosed with cancer . . . perhaps the world will be annihilated in a nuclear war. But these worries are usually only momentary. For all intents and purposes, I carry on daily life as though what is happening will go on forever. I just never let the fact of death upset this ongoing and vague sense of my immortality."

Everyday immortality occurs less as a persistent idea but more as something imprinted into our daily routines and enacted within the course of daily life. It is not directly thought about because to do so opens up the possibility of uncovering it as false and absurd. It is more enacted or performed in the way we conduct ourselves throughout the course of daily pursuits. This is why evasion practices around talking or thinking about my-death play such a vital role. They make it less likely that the pretense of immortality will be revealed, and, accordingly, the activities associated with performing a life that goes on forever become firmly embedded.

So, ideas that shield us from the reality of my-death can play a significant role in maintaining our collective sense of strategic immortality. These ideas come in many shapes and sizes. For example, the idea of our souls persisting beyond death helps to de-emphasize the significance of my-death. If

I understand my soul to reside somewhere after death, then my-death can be viewed as a transition point rather than posing any other more fundamental challenges to my being. Similarly, the idea of my consciousness playing a small part in a larger universal or cosmic consciousness helps draw attention away from the importance of my-death.[28] But ideas are not the only strategy we use to facilitate everyday evasion of my-death. Culture and language provide an array of common symbols and conventions that also create a space for the pretense of immortality.

As the afternoon sun arced slowly closer to the treetops, Brenda stretched forward and poured out more wine. "Here, Stan, have another glass."

"Ooh, thank you. I'm beginning to feel it seeping through my brain. Why stop now?"

As he sipped the cool liquid, he closed his eyes and pointed his face directly into the warm rays of the sun.

"It's funny, Stan, the way we tiptoe around when talking to others about someone's death; 'specially when speaking to a loved-one."

"Yes, that's right. It's common for people to say how sorry they are to hear about someone 'passing on,' as in, 'It's so sad to hear about Uncle Joe passing'; as though he's moved on somewhere else . . . like he's moved house or moved to another country."

"Or what about when someone says, 'We lost Uncle Joe last night?' It's as though he's shifted somewhere we don't know about and that, if we look hard enough, we might just be able to find him again."

"He's lost, and he might be found," reflected Stan. "This talk must be very confusing to children."

"Yes. If my niece heard that, she would be more than likely to start searching for him," observed Brenda with a faint giggle. "All right, what about when we talk of Uncle Joe 'falling asleep.' I've seen this on gravestones: so-and-so 'fell asleep' on the twenty-first of July, 1933. It's a bit like saying someone turned off the lights in his mind and now he's asleep or unconscious."

"Um, that is common," noted Stan, "and sometimes it's given a religious flavor by saying he's 'resting in peace' or he's attained 'eternal rest.'"

"And there's the funny ones that make light of the whole business. Like, Uncle Joe's 'pushing up daisies,' he's 'kicked the bucket,' or he's 'given up the ghost.'"

"Yes, there's lots of those."

Brenda bent forward and suspended the wine bottle over Stan's empty glass. "Another?"

"Ah no. I'm feeling a bit too light-headed."

She leaned back to watch the sun disappearing behind the trees. "But I suppose we often play down or make light of death to soften any reference to dying in case loved ones are really struggling with accepting it as a death. It cushions the blow. I find myself talking this way all day."

"I'm not sure it's only about protecting others. I think we also do it to shelter ourselves."

"Ah, yeah, I guess it does help me day to day to pretend that it's not going to happen."

Metaphors and euphemisms of death, such as going to sleep, turning off the light, or moving to another place, add to our repertoire of my-death evasion strategies.[29] They provide additional assistance in our task of keeping focused on daily realities and in avoiding the paralyzing dilemmas posed by my-death. In this way they help us move forward inside the protective bubble of everyday immortality.

Bursting the Bubble

Despite day-to-day playing down, ignoring, or denying of the reality of death, the specter of death in its various guises stands resolutely and uncompromisingly in front of each of us as we proceed through life. As Herman Melville in his novel *Moby-Dick* asserted,

> *All men live enveloped in whale-lines. All are born with halters around their necks; but it is only when caught in the swift, sudden turn of death, that mortals realize the silent, subtle, ever-present perils of life. And if you be a philosopher, though seated in the whale-boat, you would not at heart feel one whit more of terror, than though seated before your evening fire with a poker, and not a harpoon, by your side.[30]*

Every now and then, the bubble we surround ourselves with, this daily pretense of immortality, is prodded and poked, and occasionally the thin membrane that holds it together collapses. At such moments we turn and face my-death, in all its unfathomable ruthlessness, and, in doing so, its close and immediate presence is revealed.

Mandy was sitting in the armchair by the fireplace in the living room browsing through a cookbook and wondering what to have for dinner. Her research ended abruptly when Leo marched into the room, flopped onto the couch, and leaned forward with his chin cradled in his hands.

"Leo, your face. It's as white as a sheet. Are you okay?"

Leo looked up and frowned but chose not to answer.

"Has something happened?"

"Ah, yes." He leaned back and sighed. "It was close, Mom, real close."

Mandy put the magazine down and leaned forward. "You look all shook up." She stared at him with a concerned expression. "Tell me what happened. . . . Were you nearly in an accident?"

"Not exactly," he replied with a reluctant tone. "Okay, okay. I guess it won't hurt to tell you." He leaned back in the couch and stared back at his mother. "Well, earlier, as the sun was setting, I was walking along the cliffs around the edge of the quarry. You know that path along the top?"

"Yes," Mandy frowned. "You really shouldn't go up there, particularly in bad light. But I guess it's safe enough, at least with the fence a bit back from the edge."

"Um, yeah. But suddenly I thought I saw an animal, a rabbit or a hare, scamper over the cliff, so, I climbed the fence to take a closer look. I couldn't see anything, so I turned and tried to head back toward the fence. But, since I was standing on some damp mossy rock, as I turned I slipped and my legs ended up dangling off the edge. . . ."

"Shit," Mandy responded involuntarily.

"As I fell onto the ground, I managed to grab hold of some tussocky grass, which I held onto with all my might. There I was, lying there, my hands on the grass and my legs off the edge."

"Oh, my God, you could have fallen."

"No, no. I was all right," Leo reassured his mother. "Once I grabbed the grass I knew I was okay. But . . . but what really affected me was the suddenness of it all. A few moments before I'd been walking along wondering what to do on the weekend; next minute, I'm lying right on the edge of destruction. The two totally different moments were so close together. It made me think that at any point in my life death can declare itself; it is really only a hair's breath away."

Leo was shocked at how abruptly the prospect of my-death was able to assert itself in his mind. One moment he was thinking about what lay ahead in the next few days, as he normally did, and the next moment his life, his mind, and his future all appeared vulnerable and at risk.

The near-at-hand nature of my-death is not limited to close calls with dying. A wide range of other events and sources have the capacity to stimulate and, at times, trigger awareness of my-death.[31] Art and literature is one source that has the potential to evoke a sense of the fragility of life and the importance of one's own mortality. For example, the New England poet Emily Dickinson created verse filled with direct and figurative references to my-death.[32] Many artists have grappled with themes and images that highlight the subtleties and complexities of death, from Ancient Egyptian death murals, to Greek funeral vases, to paintings by Botticeli, Caravaggio, Goya, Klimt, Hirst, and many, many more.[33] Similarly, film writers and directors draw on a vast array of images, symbols, and metaphors of death.[34] Besides works of art, another space in which my-death awareness might be activated is in nature environments such as viewing a sunset, observing animals dying, or staring into an abyss.[35] Moreover, such awareness can occur in the most unlikely places; for instance Grant and Wade-Benzoni (2009) examined the various ways in which death awareness is triggered in the workplace by events such as dangerous tasks and retirements.[36]

These cues and triggers interact in complex ways with different aspects of death.[37] Sometimes the focus is on dying, sometimes on other-death, sometimes on my-death, and sometimes on all three of these simultaneously. When Leo told his mother about his close call with death, he focused mainly on the risk of dying. But this was only a partial disclosure. Another layer, which he did not talk to her about, concerned how this experience revealed more intimate aspects of his ongoing relationship to my-death.

After Mandy went to bed, Leo crossed into the kitchen to pour himself a glass of milk. As he entered, he could see Brenda under the lamp on the kitchen table writing something into an exercise book. He carried his glass over to the table and sat down opposite her.

"Hi, 'spose you're writing something about your patients?"

Brenda looked up and stated sternly, "Your Mom asked me not to speak to you about my job, or about depressing or morose topics, particularly about death."

"Ah, she worries too much. Besides, she's really phobic about dying and all that; reckons it's morbid. I told her she's got it all wrong."

"Okay, but let's just keep her happy and stay off such topics."

Leo nodded vaguely but continued on. "Brenda, you know how suddenly things can happen to you that change your whole view about what life is about?"

"Hmm, yes. But what are you getting at?"

"Well, this evening I was walking along the top of the cliff by the quarry, and, for some reason, I climbed over the fence, walked to the edge, and stared down. I was right on the edge; one step further and I would have fallen hundreds of feet to be shattered apart on the rocks below." He gulped down some of his milk. "As I stood there imagining it happening, a kind of shudder went through my body and I felt myself being strangely pulled even closer to the edge. It was a weird feeling; as if I was transfixed by the possibility of falling. I even stuck my toes out over the edge." He wiped the milk off his upper lip. "It would have taken nothing; one tiny step and it would've all been over."

"My God, were you really thinking of killing yourself?"[38]

"I wasn't running away from anything, if that's what you mean. More I felt I was being drawn toward something; like I was somehow being mysteriously enticed into finding out what it might mean if I jumped: What would happen? Where would I go? Would it be the end of everything?" He paused to drink down some of his milk. "It was all so close and tangible; it would have been nothing to go there."

"Okay, so what was it that made you look at things differently?"

"I guess the pull I felt to jump highlighted how close I am to my own death. It's always there . . . a constant possibility, a constant companion . . . and it sits there next to me at every moment."

"Hmm, that's a good way of saying it: 'a constant companion.' That's the way I see it from time to time."

"Well, Brenda, we sure managed to avoid talking about morose topics, didn't we?" He smiled and finished up his milk. "See ya. I'm off to bed."

Brenda and Leo agreed that my-death can be thought of as resembling a relationship, an intimate relationship, and one that persists over the course of a lifetime. By talking this way they have relocated my-death away from the event of dying and turned it into an element or dimension of everyday living. My-death walks side by side with each of us, sometimes shadowing us, sometimes nudging us, and sometimes jumping out and startling us. The next five chapters are going to look more closely at what makes it possible for my-death to reassert its reality and become an important relationship, a "constant companion," as we stride through whatever fate determines.

Notes

1. Hesiod, in *Theogony* (John Hopkins University Press, 2004), depicts Thanatos in more negative terms.
2. For an overview of death in different religious traditions, see S. J. Rosen, ed., *Ultimate Journey: Death and Dying in the World's Major Religions* (Westport: Praeger, 2008).
3. An account of this is provided by John Kelly in *The Great Mortality: An Intimate History of the Black Death* (New York: HarperCollins, 2006).
4. An overview of the various personifications of death is provided in L. Wendell, *Encounters with Death* (New Orleans: Westgate, 1996), and details specifically on the Grim Reaper in R. Lynette, *The Grim Reaper* (Farmington Hills: KidHaven Press, 2010).
5. Elemér Hankiss, in *Fears and Symbols* (Budapest: CEU Press, 2001), argues that the symbols of our most basic fears, most importantly my-death, enable us to develop some sense of control and protection over these fears.
6. Ernest Becker, *The Denial of Death* (New York: Free Press, 2007). The book won the Pulitzer Prize for General Non-Fiction in 1974 and is quoted by as diverse figures as Woody Allen and Bill Clinton.
7. Ibid., p. 66.
8. Ibid., p. 27.
9. J. L. Brain, *The Last Taboo: Sex and the Fear of Death* (Garden City: Anchor/Doubleday, 1979). See also M. Robert and L. Tradii, "Do we deny death? I. A genealogy of death denial," *Mortality* (23:3, 247–60, 2019).
10. R. Lee, "Modernity, mortality and re-enchantment: The death taboo revisited," *Sociology* (42:4, 745–59, 2008).
11. R. McManus, *Death in a Global Age* (Basingstoke: Palgrave Macmillan, 2012) p. 28.
12. Shelly Kagan, *Death* (New Haven: Yale University Press, 2012).
13. The classic study on obedience was conducted by Stanley Milgram in 1961, in which normal people obeyed researchers into delivering what they thought were fatal shocks. A considerable body of psychological research has followed on from this, as summarized by T. Blass, ed., *Obedience to Authority* (London: Psychology Press, 1999).
14. See Lora-Jean Collett and David Lester, "The fear of death and the fear of dying," *Journal of Psychology* (72:2, 179–81, 1969).
15. Early research on this scale is summarized by David Lester in "The Collett-Lester Fear of Death Scale," in R. Neimeyer, ed., *Death Anxiety Handbook* (London: Routledge, 2015) pp. 45–60.

16. An overview of this literature is provided by R. Neimeyer, J. Wittkowski, and R. Moser, "Psychological research on death attitudes," *Death Studies* (28:4, 309–40, 2004).

17. For example, see L. S. Dickstein, "Attitudes toward death, anxiety, and social desirability," *Omega: Journal of Death and Dying* (8:4, 369–78, 1978).

18. Initially there were several researchers reporting this; for example, see B. Spilka, R. Pelligrini, and K. Dailey, "Religion, American values and death perspective," *Sociological Symposium* (1, 57–66, 1968).

19. See K. G. Magni, "The fear of death," in A. Godin, ed., *Death and Presence: The Psychology of Death and Afterlife* (Brussels: Lumen Vitae, 1972) pp. 125–38.

20. This multidimensional scale consisting of thirty-one questions was developed by V. Florian and S. Kravetz, "Fear of personal death," *Journal of Personality & Social Psychology* (44, 600–7, 1983), and consisted of six subscales that included "loss of self-fulfilment," "transcendental consequences," and "self-annihilation."

21. See R. H. Aday, "Belief in afterlife and death anxiety," *OMEGA-Journal of Death and Dying* (15:1, 67–75, 1985) p. 185. This idea of a more fundamental level of connection is also argued by A. Lazar, "Fear of personal death as a predictor of motivation for religious behavior," *Review of Religious Research* (48:2, 179–89, 2006).

22. A. M. Downey, "Relationship of religiosity to death anxiety of middle-aged males," *Psychological Reports* (54:3, 811–22, 1984).

23. See P. Wink and J. Scott, "Does religiousness buffer against the fear of death and dying in late adulthood?" *Journals of Gerontology* (60b:4, 207–14, 2005).

24. See L. Ellis and E. Wahab, "Religiosity and fear of death," *Review of Religious Research* (55:1, 149–89, 2013).

25. See J. Jong et al., "The religious correlates of death anxiety," *Religion, Brain & Behavior* (8:1, 4–20, 2018) p. 17.

26. For more on fear, see P. L. Gower, *Psychology of Fear* (New York: Nova Science, 2004).

27. The social and cultural dimensions of fear are discussed in Frank Furedi, *Culture of Fear Revisited: Risk-Taking and the Morality of Low Expectation, Fourth Edition* (London: Continuum, 2006).

28. The idea of cosmic and universal consciousness was championed more than a century ago by writers such as Evelyn Underhill, *Mysticism: A Study in the Nature and Development of Man's Spiritual Consciousness* (London: Methuen, 1911) and Richard Bucke, *Cosmic Consciousness: A Study in the Evolution of the Human Mind* (New York: Dutton & Co., 1923, 1901). Similarly, according to Hindu faith, death is seen as a natural part of the cycle of life, death, and afterlife which together form part of the path to perfect oneness with God. See Shyam Ghosh, *Hindu Concept of Life and Death: As Portrayed in Vedas, Brahmanas, Aranyakas, Upanisads* (New Delhi: Munshiram Manoharlal Publishers, 2002).

29. More complete coverage of common metaphors of death is provided by L. Ross and H. Pollio, "Metaphors of death," *Omega: Journal of Death and Dying* (23:4, 291–307, 1991).

30. Herman Melville, *Moby-Dick* (New York: Dover, 2003, 1851) p. 232. Much has been written about the great white whale as a symbol or metaphor of personal mortality. For example, see this discussed by James Grove in "Melville's vision of death

in Moby-Dick: Stepping away from the 'snug sofa,'" *New England Quarterly* (52:2, 177–96, 1979).

31. This is discussed in L. Harvell and G. Nisbeth, eds., *Denying Death: An Interdisciplinary Approach to Terror Management Theory* (New York: Routledge, 2016), where they pointed out how awareness of my-death is not confined to frightening incidents. Terror management theory is more fully discussed in the first section of Chapter 11.

32. J. Deppman provides a detailed account of Dickinson's ways of discussing mortality in "Dickinson, death, and the sublime," *The Emily Dickinson Journal* (9:1, 1–20, 2000).

33. For a more general discussion, see Chris Townsend, *Art and Death* (London: I. B. Tauris, 2008).

34. For a collection of essays about death in films, see D. Sullivan and J. Greenberg, eds., *Death in Classic and Contemporary Film* (New York: Palgrave Macmillan, 2013).

35. Some of the natural events that can promote death awareness are discussed by Irving Yalom in *Staring at the Sun: Overcoming the Terror of Death* (San Francisco: Jossey-Bass, 2010).

36. See A. Grant and K. Wade-Benzoni, "The hot and cool of death awareness at work," *Academy of Management Review* (34:4, 600–32, 2009).

37. For an overview of the complexity of our awareness and fear of death, see M. Mikulincer and V. Florian, "The complex mulifaceted nature of the fear of personal death," in A. Tomer et al., eds., *Existential and Spiritual Issues in Death Attitudes* (New York: Laurence Erlbaum, 2013).

38. Here, Brenda is referencing the topic of suicide, a big topic with many aspects to consider, and, while its study is dominated by considerations of dying and other-death, it has some connections to conceptions of my-death. Ever since Émile Durkheim's classic book, *Suicide: A Study in Sociology* (Taylor & Francis, e-book, 2005, 1951), suicidology has expanded but surprisingly little attention has focused on my-death except for some explorations of the existential aspects of suicide as summarized by Israel Orbach, "Existentialism and suicide," in Tomer et al. (2013).

5

A Constant Companion

Let's pick up on Leo's passing comment when he referred to my-death as "a constant companion." What he appeared to be suggesting, and Brenda recognized it immediately, was that, despite the blurring and obscuring of my-death with the dying of other people and despite common evasion of thinking about it, my-death still manages to insinuate its presence into our daily lives. We somehow continue to connect from time to time with it in some form, even if it is only a vague awareness in the back of our minds. The Lithuanian-French thinker Emmanuel Levinas (2000) recognized this when he claimed:

> One does not know, one cannot be present at, one's annihilation . . .; this is the case not only because of the nothingness that cannot be given as a thematizable event. . . . My relationship with death is a nonknowledge on dying itself, a nonknowledge that is nevertheless not an absence of relationship.[1]

Levinas developed his own theories on how we might connect with my-death as "nonknowledge." The impossibility of being able to directly know or speak about my-death does not preclude other ways of connecting and thereby of forming an ongoing relationship. However, this does require a shift in how we see both the nature of the connection and that which does the connecting: namely, the self.

Relational Identity

The nature of selfhood can be approached from a range of angles. The most common and familiar way is to view the self as an individual particle located in one time and place and made up of a range of properties and attributes.[2] Who I am is this thing here, this thing in a body, this presence in a mind, somehow vaguely located in my brain or perhaps somewhere at the intersection of my senses. Wherever I go, it moves with me; with whomever I interact, it is this that they point to and identify as me, and, whichever relationships I enter, it is this individual me-self that occupies at least one pole in that arrangement. Moreover I can project this individualistic frame onto other people. I can see them also as discrete autonomous units, self-contained objects with distinct bodies and minds, moving about within a shared environment, connecting and disconnecting much like balls bouncing off each other across a billiard table. I can also make sense of their behavior through my knowledge of the attributes which are contained and travel about inside them. Similar to the way I judge the movement of a ball by attributes such as mass, inertia, and its angle of movement, so I make judgments of the behaviors of other people based on my knowledge of contained attributes such as intelligence, character, beliefs, and motivations. What both the body-particle (bio-medical) and mind-particle (psychological) interpretations have in common is a thorough commitment to the nature of selfhood residing firmly with this autonomous individualized self.

However, there is another, significantly different way of approaching the nature of selfhood. Instead of viewing the self as pertaining to a specific location, the place where the body houses the mind, the self can be viewed as interfused through the multitude of meaningful relationships that surround each person and within which identity is forged.

Brenda heard Winston barking the moment she knocked on Stan's door. She had brought some fruit and cheese for Stan to snack on, but her real motive was to speak about the difficulties she was having with Mandy.

"Come in, come on in," beckoned Stan. "You're most welcome." He took the fruit and led her into his kitchen, where he put the kettle on and proceeded to wash the grapes and place them on a platter. As he cut up the cantaloupe, he asked, "So how's it going next door?"

"I dunno, Stan. Whenever I'm with Mandy, I feel I'm walking on eggshells. Don't get me wrong, I like her, and I think we could get along, but she's constantly questioning my approach to things, particularly the way I relate to Leo. It's got so bad that I'm avoiding Leo in case she misinterprets what we're talking about."

"Ah, she's like that," he said as he placed the melon slices on the platter and the cheese with a knife on a cheese-board. "I've known her since she was a child. She's always been a rather uptight person."

"Hmm." Brenda paused and stared momentarily at Stan. "I'm sorry, Stan, I can't really accept that. People get uptight for particular reasons. I don't think she's naturally uptight; just that circumstances have driven her to be like that."

"Well she sure gets worked up about little things," said Stan as he beckoned her over to sit at his kitchen table. "Coffee?"

"Yes, okay; with a dash of milk; no sugar." She sat watching Stan pouring the coffee into two colorful mugs. "Look, I stopped some time ago looking at people around me as permanently fixed or trapped in particular personalities. In the past, to my shame, I used to talk about this person being aggressive and this person being steadfast, and this person being caring. But now, I don't see people I know as captured by their qualities."

Stan walked over with the two mugs and sat down at the table opposite her. "I'm not sure, but in my experience people tend to behave in similar ways right through their lives."

"That might well be . . . ," said Brenda, staring in silence into a space above Stan's head. "I remember some time ago, in my early years of nursing, I used to think of myself, my identity, as belonging to this place here," she drew out her hands and brought them close her chest, "this thing here, this flesh and blood," she touched the top of her head, "this mind. This is from where my consciousness is located and where I as a person reside."

"Yeah, that's right. That *is* where you are," he copied her previous hand motion toward his own chest, "and this *is* where I am."

"But as I cared for more people, particularly when I moved to nursing those at the end of their lives, my views slowly changed. I began seeing each person more as a product of their relationships. The process of dying slowly strips you back to bare essentials and highlights what's most important. And what's important to most people are their relationships. Not just their relationships to their loved ones, but their relationships to their environment—trees, hills, rivers—and their relationships to whatever form of spirituality they prefer, and to their passions—their hobbies, their achievements, their talents. All these relationships provide them with the platform for knowing who they are."

The shift from an individualistic understanding of the self to a relational view opens up a range of different ways of thinking about who we are as people.[3] The focus moves from viewing the self as primarily a discrete particle to viewing it more as an intersection point situated within a complex web of relationships. Instead of emphasizing the qualities and attributes we possess, the emphasis shifts toward the types of the relationships we inhabit.

The shift toward a relational perspective has prompted and, in turn, found support in a range of academic movements. The streams of activity include various schools of French philosophy, large parts of North American sociology and anthropology, and a lively network in British social psychology, as well as a range of activities in social geography, culture and gender studies, and literary criticism. To touch briefly on one of the early figures, the Viennese-born American sociologist Alfred Schutz managed through his teaching and writing to coax other sociologists to begin looking more closely at how a person's situation in everyday life affects his or her experience as a whole. In his book *The Phenomenology of the Social World* he connected the domain of personal meaning with the domain of action and explored how these are constituted through the interaction of experience and the social world.[4] Sociologists influenced by his work (students such as Peter Berger and contemporaries such as Harold Garfinkel) took on board his shift from an emphasis on overarching structural processes (such as "class" and "market") to an emphasis on the experience of social involvements and went on to develop theories and methods that examined how value and identity are often derived from the particularities of specific situations.[5] Those who followed, and many from other social theory traditions, have helped sketch the fine detail of how people experience their situatedness in everyday life and the complex dynamics of social interrelations. The shift in thinking has contributed to a range of important theories of identity which include relational identity theory in management studies, social identity theory in psychology, and symbolic interactionist theory in sociology.[6]

The interest of social scientists in relational interpretations of selfhood spilled over into studies of health and well-being, particularly those associated with community development, youth well-being, and mental health. A key person in this transmission was the psychologist Urie Bronfenbrenner (1979) whose socio-ecological theory had wide implications for how we understand the strength and resilience of both individuals and communities.[7] Instead of viewing a person's strength in terms of accumulated resources located in the individual, strength is seen more as a product of the quality of relationships in the nexus of interconnections that surround a person in the course of daily life.[8] For instance, socio-ecological theory has played an important role in shifting the emphasis of research with youth at risk from a focus on what is going wrong with individuals (such as distorted thinking, mental health issues, and drug use) to asking what is going right and what promotes strength in terms of their social contexts. Indeed, the study of youth well-being has switched dramatically from deficit understandings to asset explanations, with a young person's connectedness to their social world—home, school, and friends—as the primary focus.[9]

However, interpretations of the self in terms of isolated attribute-bearing individuals remain deeply ingrained in how we understand why people do what they do. It is still difficult to persuade others of the merits of interpreting selfhood in terms of relationships.

Brenda and Stan's conversation was interrupted by a tapping on the kitchen door. Winston scrambled to attention and trotted over to the door, barking at the intruder. Stan followed and, pulling Winston gently back by his collar, opened the door. "Ah, Leo, good to see you. Come and join us in a coffee and a chat."

Leo settled himself at the table while Stan poured him out a mug of coffee. "So, what have you two been discussing?"

"Hmm, it's a bit hard to explain," said Stan. "Brenda reckons your relationships make up more of you than the qualities of you as a person," he explained as he resumed his seat, "but I'm not so sure."

"Yes, Stan, but I'm saying more than that," clarified Brenda. "I'm saying that relationships provide the raw material, the substance with which we build up a sense of who we are."

"Okay, I've moved through lots of relationships, big and small, positive and negative, significant and not-so-significant," stated Stan, "but there's still this me-person, with all my qualities, that does this moving. This self of mine just keeps learning and adapting and becoming this essential 'I' that I am."

"That's right," agreed Leo, "I am an individual; I have this total sense of being what I am."

"Ah ha," said Brenda, "you are a distinct individual; a unique person with a unique combination of attributes. But let's just look a little closer at what might be meant by 'attributes.' Say, for instance, you were to claim you're 'a caring person.' This quality, 'caring,' where does it come from? Surely it doesn't come from within? No, it has been patterned into who you are according the way your relationships have unfolded."

"Yeah, that's kind of obvious," commented Leo, "but it doesn't follow that who I am can be reduced to my relationships."

"Okay, try this one out," offered Brenda, feeling a bit pressured. "Let's say you were to somehow take off from Earth and end up landing on

Mars—don't know how you'd do it, but just imagine it's possible. You're walking along a dusty path, and you amble past several local Martians who each look at you strangely. To them you look a bit weird, and they are curious about what makes you tick. So each of them asks, 'Who are you?' How might you respond to such a question?"

"Hmm. Unlikely to happen," responded Leo, "and if it did I wouldn't have much to go on. But I guess what I'd do is try to describe the type of person I am. 'I'm a thoughtful person,' 'I enjoy talking with people,' 'I can be a bit abrupt at times.'"

"Sure, in response you could talk about your personal attributes, or . . ." Brenda paused to check Leo and Stan were following, " . . . or, rather than talking about attributes, you could talk about the various relationships that define who you are: 'I have two children,' 'I work as a lawyer in a patents office,' 'I play poker regularly with my closest friends.' See, instead of my qualities and attributes, I'm now talking about my relationships. For Martians, this is surely far easier to grasp than talking about abstract concepts such as being generous or being impatient—concepts which are derived from the way we engage in relationships anyway."

Brenda was promoting a relational view by acknowledging individual attributes as important, but only as part of the picture of identity formation. She was arguing that personal attributes are, on the whole, derived from what is observed within relationships; that the real substance of identity comes from how we understand ourselves within our interconnected social worlds.

My-Death Relationality

One way to approach my-death is to view it as a constantly present attribute belonging to the self; as though my-death is an ingredient in what it means for me to be alive. This "me," this central ego, carries my-death along with it as one of the components that contributes to what it means to be an individual just as I carry my personality, my body, even my mind around with me. But what would happen if my-death was shifted from an individualistic to a social understanding of the self? How would this change how we might think about my-death?

The repositioning of my-death from an individualistic perspective to viewing it as one relationship among other relationships shifts it from being seen as a free-floating, vague presence and places it in among the fluid and dynamic processes that characterize most of our relationships. For example, the dynamism of a close family relationship—such as a marriage—occurs at several levels: first, it is bidirectional, with my partner helping to define my identity just as I help to define his or her identity; second, it shifts and changes over time, with some periods of strong intimacy and other periods of reduced closeness; and, third, it involves variations in power, with either party feeling more or less in control at different times. Now, each of these can be applied to a relational view of my-death: first, it can be seen as bidirectional, both because it is incorporated into my sense of self and because I can influence how it is perceived; second, as our four characters have illustrated, relationships to my-death shift and change over time, sometimes flipping dramatically from something benign to something terrifying or vice versa; and, third, the balance of power in the relationship can shift my-death from being seen as life-enhancing to being seen as totally dominating and oppressive.

Brenda noticed that Stan was staring with a fixed expression into vacant space. He seemed deeply immersed in his own thoughts. "So, Stan, tell us what you've been thinking?"

"Ah, I'm. . . ." his gaze snapped back onto Brenda and Leo sitting at the table. "I'm thinking over what you've just been saying and wondering how it might apply to what we were talking about last week; you know, to thoughts about our own deaths."

"Hmm, Stan, that's an interesting question." Brenda paused and glanced across at Leo. "Now listen Leo, your mother has made it very clear she doesn't approve of us talking about morbid topics like death. I don't want to upset her."

"Ah, look, she's overreacting. I talk about this stuff all the time with my friends. It's not going to upset me. She really doesn't need to know."

"I'm not comfortable with that."

"Please, don't worry, I'm fine with it."

"Okay, as long as you don't tell her." Brenda was willing to proceed because she was intrigued by the direction of the conversation, and she wanted to explore Stan's idea further. She was more than a little surprised at the conceptual leap he was making. "So, Stan, let's see where this takes us. If you look at your own death as an ongoing relationship, what do you think that implies?"

"Well, I guess it implies it's always there and, that . . . I guess, depending on the way I enter this relationship . . . that will determine what it means for my identity." He paused to consider what he had just said. "It also suggests I'm always in this relationship, whether I turn my back on it and ignore it . . . or whether I choose to face it and incorporate it into my life; it's always there."

"I like that," commented Brenda, "'It's always there.'" She smiled. "I'd add, 'whether you like it or not.' It's always there, a constant presence."

Leo was listening but remained unconvinced about what they were asserting. "Yes, but surely my death is something very personal. It's not an outside relationship; it belongs to my innermost depths." He took a large gulp from his half-cooled coffee. "Besides, out of anything else in my life, my death belongs totally to me: nobody else can share it, nobody else can do it for me. It's the one thing that I and only I can do for myself!"

"Yes, I agree," said Stan with a smile spreading across his wrinkled face. "But if I understand Brenda correctly, relationships don't always need to be between two people, or even between two easily identified objects. I have many relationships that are important to me but involve more abstract things like my future, or my past, or my reputation, or my belief in principles such as national pride or academic freedom; these are complex and abstract relationships, but that doesn't make them any less important. For instance, my relationship to my future matters to me a great deal; I spend a lot of time thinking about that."

Stan and Brenda both recognized how our interconnections with the world involve more than simple object-to-object or self-to-object relationships. Many of our relationships involve connections to abstract and ethereal entities such as ethical principles or future ambitions. Accordingly, even though my-death is difficult to point to or to think about or to locate, it does not follow that we cannot see ourselves having a relationship to it. It could join that vast array of solid and abstract objects we use to build up our sense of self.

"You know," commented Brenda, staring down at her half-filled mug, "I can see how looking at ourselves in terms of relationships changes the nature of how we see death altogether. For example, when someone close dies, it's not the absence of this discrete person that matters; rather, it's the way this changes relationships. I see this every day."

"You mean," clarified Leo, "if I was married and my partner died, I would be constantly interacting with the spaces in which she is no longer present. In this way I would continue in some kind of relationship with her?"

"Yes, when she was alive you would be participating in a continual series of relationships not only with her but with everything surrounding her . . . and everything surrounding you both. You come home and sit eating your meal with her at the table, then you sit together on the sofa watching television, then you lie together in bed. At each point you and your context are both situated in a series of shared relationships. Then, when she dies, that which previously surrounded her is still present, so you, in a sense continue to relate to her but with the center of what you identified as 'her' as no longer present."

"Hmm, this is tricky," admitted Leo. "So, you mean, when I come home, my recently dead wife remains as a present absence?"

"Yes, that's it. Her absence sits in the middle of a concentric ring of relationships that you are still connected to. She hasn't disappeared. She is still present, and absent, at the table, on the sofa, and in the bed. You remain living with her relational presence. And it stays like that for a long time because it's not just your relationship to her absence that matters, but the relationship of others to her absence as well as your relationship to them."

Stan had been listening intently and decided to join in. "That's precisely what happened to me when my wife died all those years ago. For years I came home to sit eating my dinner opposite her absence, then her absence was hovering there next to me whenever I went for a walk or did some shopping; again, there it was next to me whenever I went out to dinner. Even today, I still have this nagging sense of her presence in so many of the places we shared."

"Okay," said Leo, "but you're talking about other people dying here. How might you apply it to your own death?"

"Well, it's the same," stated Brenda confidently. "If I see my own death as a relational possibility that is kind of present but present as an absence and in a similar way to departed loved-ones, I can see myself in a continual relationship with it."

The trio were talking through some conceptually difficult territory. With the death of another person, the presence and, to some extent, the absence of the person involved can be located within the relationships that comprise one's social world. Prior to the person dying, the relationship is easily seen as a connection between one person and another, and, when that person dies, his or her absent position within the nexus of relationships can still be located; the absence is surrounded by the many relationships that were previously active, so it is something that can still be referenced even though the original object has disappeared. But, as Leo quite rightly pointed out, this is not so easily applied to one's own death. In pursuing a relationship to my-death, it is very unclear to what object we might be connecting.

Here lies the crux of the problem for pursuing a relationship with my-death. As discussed in Chapter 3, my-death is unthinkable and unspeakable, which also makes it untouchable. It cannot be seen as an absence in the same way it is applied to another person's death because, as I am alive, it is not viable to view myself as an absence. At the point of my death, all this will be put at risk because my consciousness comes to an end, and, accordingly, I would then lack any sort of position from which to observe my absence. So, by what means might I conceive of entering a relationship to my-death?

Leo was feeling a little annoyed, even ganged up on. Stan appeared to have crossed over to back Brenda's position. His youthful skepticism no longer seemed to have currency. "Okay, okay, I'll go along with it. I mean I'll accept, for now, the idea of approaching my own death as a relationship."

"Good," said Stan smiling benevolently. "But Leo, I'm mindful of our conclusion a week ago that there's no way of really thinking about one's own death. You remember? It's beyond knowing, thinking, or speaking."

"Well, that's my point," claimed Leo. "That's what makes my death completely untouchable. How can you have a relationship with something you can't think or talk about?"

"Yes, it's frustrating," added Brenda. "I have this sense that my death is there; it's always somehow with me, but I can't locate it. It's like trying to form a relationship with a shadow, or a rainbow, or some other elusive image."

"But, as we were just saying," said Stan, "it is possible to have relationships with vague objects like my future or my legacy; why not my death?" He paused for effect, then gulped down the remainder of his coffee. "But, I admit, not being able to talk or think about it does make it more difficult."

"Hmm, yes, it sure does," agreed Brenda.

"I think what's missing," offered Stan, "is having some way of grasping and holding on to my death; without a point of contact it just slips away. What's needed is something like a provisional handle, or a hook, that your mind might be able to link up with."

"Okay, so let's think a bit about that," suggested Leo. "What are the types of relationships that people manage to have with their own mortality?"

"Hmm, that's interesting . . . ," muttered Brenda. "I guess one common relationship is no relationship at all. Seems to me many people are quite happy to ignore it. They carry on totally disinterested until it hits them in the face when they are told they have a terminal illness."

Stan frowned, "I'd say that's how it looks from the outside, but many of those same people do think about it from time to time and it frightens them. I was one of them; I pretended it didn't bother me, but deep down I was terrified by it, so I made a point of not thinking about it."

"Okay, so . . . ," Leo paused to collect his thoughts. "So we have some people not thinking about it, others who think about it but avoid it because it frightens them, but there's another group who realize death is inevitable but just don't know what to make of it, so they end up feeling frustrated. I reckon we're all going through a bit of that."

"I guess," added Stan, "many of those are attracted to death in indirect ways, they feel drawn to various representations of death, often in the form of death imagery or death symbols, maybe embedded in painting or poetry or theater. But I don't think these images are sufficient to form a proper relationship. We need something more; something more stable that we can grab hold of."

"Like a concept or a theory," suggested Brenda.

"Yes," agreed Stan, "a provisional idea which acts as a helpful device that allows me to construct a relationship around the nothingness of death."

This discussion sets up the central challenge for the following five chapters. For there to be a relationship to an object as elusive, insubstantial, and unthinkable as my-death, we require some sort of provisional handhold that allows our minds to reach out and grasp onto something to act as an object with which to form a relationship. Without it, a meaningful relationship would struggle to take shape. What is required is some sort of conceptual mechanism or helpful device that enables a relationship to be conceived.

Enabling Frames

For the purposes of this book, I am going to refer to these helpful devices as "enabling frames."[10] First, they are *enabling* because, rather than attempting to describe the nature of reality, their core function is to help make what would otherwise be unfathomable, fathomable. They provide an anchoring point to focus the mind on where and how a relationship with my-death could be located. Second, they are *frames* because, as with other studies of framing in fields such as political studies and marketing, they involve a coordinated collection of interlinking communication strategies that help bring into focus a particular way of looking at things.

The key role that communication strategies play in generating enabling frames links them in many important ways to the field of rhetoric. Throughout the long history of rhetoric, attention has focused primarily on the way something is expressed rather than what is expressed, but, in doing so, rhetoricians are careful to avoid claiming that rhetoric could ever replace having something to say; they contend merely that the manner of delivery plays an important part in determining how a message will be received.[11] In ancient Greek and Roman times, rhetoric—including oratory—was understood as the study of persuasive communication and was seen as one of the three cornerstones of knowledge.[12] At the center of this field of study lay those elements in a communication which convey senses over and above its literal meaning. These elements were identified as specific rhetorical devices or "tropes," and, right from the start, rhetoricians devoted considerable time and energy to classifying and labeling these devices because, once they are appropriately classified, they can be effectively deployed.[13] They found these devices could operate at both micro and macro levels within a communication. The more micro-level devices include *phoneme regularities*, such as repeated sounds (e.g., "the cat is on the mat"), and the *missing out of expected content*, such as ellipses and unfinished sentences. At the more macro-level, devices include larger conceptual references, such as *metaphor* (e.g., "a pregnant pause"), and overall ways of organizing the whole communications, such as using different forms of narrative.[14]

From the seventeenth century into the enlightenment of the twentieth century, a change was taking place. Writers were starting to view the noble art of rhetoric in less positive terms. Prominent thinkers, such as Immanuel Kant, Francis Bacon, and Auguste Comte, were expressing concern about the polluting influence rhetoric was having on moral behavior and on the integrity of knowledge. For instance, Kant referred to oratory as "the art of playing for one's own purpose upon the weaknesses of men . . . and merits no respect whatever."[15] By the early nineteenth century, the tide of academic opinion had definitely turned, and rhetoric had deteriorated from a dynamic and developing discipline into a static cataloguing of figures of speech.[16] By the end of the nineteenth century, Thomas de Quincey (2010, 1897) was declaring:

> *The age of Rhetoric, like that of Chivalry, has passed amongst forgotten things; and the rhetorician can have no more chance for returning than the rhapsodist of early Greece or the troubadour of romance.*[17]

Despite this pronouncement, the twentieth and twenty-first centuries witnessed a steadily growing resurgence of academic interest in rhetoric. Supporters of the revival argued that nonliteral or rhetorical content of a communication does not necessarily oppose or obscure its rational content; instead, rhetorical aspects can be understood to bring into view or help highlight the rationality of what is being stated. The modern revival of rhetoric—frequently referred to as the "new rhetoric"[18]—has spread through disciplines in the humanities and the social sciences, often with a particular focus on the use of narrative and metaphor. This revival has also led to renewed interest in classifying and recording the use of rhetorical devices[19] in such diverse forms of communication as advertising, psychotherapy, political speeches, and legal arguments.[20]

More recently, rhetoric has been applied to the use of frames in the media, particularly as regards political discourses.[21] From this literature, several important features of frames have been identified. First, a frame is built around a central idea regarding how one object or domain relates to another object or domain. In order for a listener to respond to a frame, he or she needs to be familiar with this central idea, otherwise other embellishments will have little effect.[22] For example, a listener needs to appreciate the idea of "free speech" before metaphors like "cover up" or "smoke screen" make any sense. Second, the central idea in one frame is elevated above other competing frames through the use of rhetorical devices. As with all rhetoric, the three most effective devices are metaphor, associative linkages (*metonymy*), and categorical linkages (*synecdoche*).[23] For example, the central idea of "restricting immigration" might be reinforced using the metaphor of a plague or by exploiting associative linkages between people's ethnicity and terrorism. Third, each individual rhetorical device occurs within a cluster of other interlinked devices which act together to reinforce the central idea. Gamson and Modigliani (1989)[24] referred to these clusters as "interpretive packages" to emphasize the complex and coordinated way in which they tend to operate. For example, alcohol corporations make use of a variety of interlinked frames—such as "personal responsibility" and "freedom to trade"—to justify their promotion of drinking and to discourage governments from adopting public health interventions.[25]

However, much of this work on media framings appears to reinstate rhetoric as an art form seeking to manipulate people's minds and distort the truth. It misses out on the potential for rhetoric to positively enhance a meaningful utterance and to take it into territories where literal expression has difficulty venturing. These territories are particularly common when trying to communicate inner, subjective experiences. For example, when a patient tries to describe a headache to a doctor, literal descriptions—"it lasts five minutes"— convey less of what it was like than drawing on a few handy metaphors—"it's a sharp, shooting pain." Similarly, descriptions of spiritual encounters, out of necessity, call on a wide variety of rhetorical devices to capture something of what the experience was like. These typically draw on a rich combination of devices that include ellipsis (e.g., "it felt like . . ."), metaphors (e.g., "lighting up my soul"), and grammatical transpositions (e.g., "oneness," "emptiness").[26] Furthermore, these devices form strands that are wrapped around the frame's central idea and thereby provide a focus with which to form a relationship. For example, the central idea of "divinity as depth" draws on our understanding of the qualities of water to depict relationships such as the way the water's surface—or how the world appears—is contrasted what lies at depth in the water—the underlying reality—and this is further reinforced by a string of related terms such as "profound," "deeper meaning," and "beyond surface manifestations."

When we turn to the challenges of speaking about a relationship to mydeath, many of the same dilemmas crop up as occur with talking about other subjective experiences, such as pleasure and love. As highlighted in Chapter 3, trying to talk about my-death in literal ways is unlikely to achieve much. Instead, expression is forced to draw on nonliteral or figurative ways of speaking. This, accordingly, leads on to the use of enabling frames, which consist in a central idea that is then bolstered and supported by a complex of rhetorical devices.

"I'm going to put on more coffee," declared Stan as he stood up from the table, walked over to the bench, filled the kettle, and plugged it in.

Both Brenda and Leo nodded their consent to another drink. "Make mine a strong one," advised Leo.

"Won't take long," said Stan as he spooned coffee grains into the filter. "So, Leo, are you okay about us talking about your own death as an ongoing relationship?"

"Hmm, I guess . . . but I just can't see it. Even if I'm in an ongoing relationship to my own death, I can't see how it can be a real relationship like I've got with someone I care about, like a friend or someone in the family."

Stan paused as he poured boiling water into the coffee pot. "Well, there's plenty of things we have strong relationships with that aren't easy to locate or describe." He stirred the milk into the coffee, carried the mugs over to the table, then fetched a packet of cookies. "Take words like 'power' or 'love,' for instance; we don't really have a clear idea what they really mean but we still use them all the time."

"Okay, well," said Leo, "I reckon words like those are just shorthand. The concept of 'love' is just an abbreviated way to refer to the collection of all things I love, but I don't have a relationship to love itself."

"But we prattle on about love often," pointed out Stan. "We sing about it in most of our pop songs. We go on and on about the nature of love and how important it is in our lives. It's more than a collection of our various 'loves.'"

"Yes, but," said Leo, "when I talk of 'love' I think of all the people I love—like Mom and Aunty Sue—and all the activities I love—like football and hiking. These all exist, and I can relate to them. But this amorphous notion of love as a whole; I just can't imagine it as a discrete object in itself."

"Well, that's what you do," insisted Stan while sipping his hot coffee. "You cram all these experiences into one box . . . but then it takes on a life of its own and you can then build it up, give it features and character, and then it becomes an object, and that's what you have a relationship with."

"Hold on, Stan," interrupted Brenda, "I think Leo's got a point. You say love-as-a-whole exists as something we can relate to, and sure we do talk about it, like, 'love is a many splendored thing' or 'love is never saying you're sorry.' But it isn't really out there; you've constructed it, put it together; it's a convenient fiction."

"Not only that," chimed in Leo, "as a convenient fiction, it lends itself to be used in crafty ways to mislead and potentially exploit people. Look at the way our government drags 'freedom' into most of its wars."

"Look," said Stan in an annoyed tone. "It's not exploitative. You make it sound like a PR exercise; that it's just spin. I agree words like 'love' and 'freedom' are contrived and can be misused. But they also allow you to speak in ways we aren't able to otherwise."

"Okay, okay, I'm not really disagreeing," clarified Brenda concerned to prevent their conversation deteriorating into dispute. "I can see where you're leading and how we need some concepts that are contrived before we can talk of a relationship with our own death."

"Yes, so you need some way of thinking about this relationship otherwise it dissolves into everything and disperses into an abstract nothingness. Thinking in this space is like chasing butterflies, the ideas are so delicate and elusive; if you grasp them too strongly they can easily crumble, but, if you hold them too lightly, they fly away."

The challenge set for each of the next four chapters is to explore the potential of four different enabling frames to provide a handhold for reaching out and grasping onto an ongoing relationship, a constant companionship, with my-death. Without such handholds, my-death would remain elusive, invisible, and unspeakable; it would remain an impenetrable black hole from which no information is emitted and with which no connection is possible. As will be revealed, at the core of each frame sits a central idea around which reinforcing material revolves, material consisting of related concepts, supportive images, and rhetorical devices. The first enabling frame, *essential structures*, approaches my-death as an ultimate and necessary boundary in the structuring of individual existence. The second frame, *passionate suffusion*, switches to looking at my-death as something that infuses all of life and intimates its presence within all things. The third frame, *point of transition*, revisits the central idea of an afterlife, not as a way of denying my-death but as a way of embracing my-death in every moment. The fourth and final frame, *self-generative process*, seeks to avoid assumptions of outside forces powering the presence of my-death and instead visualizes a relationship created in the process of making contact.

Notes

1. E. Levinas *God, Death, and Time* (Stanford, CA: Stanford University Press, 2000) p. 19.
2. The idea of the particle self as it applies to addiction is summarized in my article, "Switching to a social approach to addiction," *International Journal of Mental Health and Addiction* (14, 86–94, 2015).
3. See F. Dépelteau, "Relational thinking: A critique of co-deterministic theories of structure and agency," *Sociological Theory* (26:1, 51–73, 2008) and K. Gergen, *Relational Being: Beyond Self and Community* (Oxford: Oxford University Press, 2009).

4. Alfred Schutz, *The Phenomenology of the Social World* (Chicago: Northwestern University Press, 1967).

5. An edited collection on issues in relational sociology is provided by C. Powell and F. Dépelteau in *Conceptualizing Relational Sociology* (New York: Palgrave Macmillan, 2013).

6. For management, see D. Sluss and B. Ashforth, "Relational identity and identification," *Academy of Management Review* (32:1, 9–32, 2007); for psychology, see J. Stets and P. Burke, "Identity theory and social identity theory," *Social Psychology Quarterly* (63:3, 224–37, 2000); for sociology, see S. Stryker, "Traditional symbolic interactionism, role theory, and structural symbolic interactionism," in J. Turner, ed., *Handbook of Sociological Theory* (Boston, MA: Springer, 2001) pp. 211–31.

7. Urie Bronfenbrenner, *The Ecology of Human Development* (Cambridge, MA: Harvard University Press, 1979). See also his edited collection, *Making Human Beings Human* (Thousand Oaks, CA: Sage, 2004).

8. David Stokol has discussed how the nexus of relationships in a community are vital for wellness in "The social ecological paradigm of wellness promotion," in M. Jamner and D. Stokols, eds., *Promoting Human Wellness: New Frontiers for Research, Practice, and Policy* (Berkeley: University of California Press, 2000).

9. This is generally referred to as "positive youth development theory." See the collection by R. Silbereisen and R. Lerner, *Approaches to Positive Youth Development* (Los Angeles: Sage, 2007).

10. In the process of choosing "enabling frames," I considered other alternatives such as "generative metaphors," as developed by D. Schön in "Generative metaphor," in A. Ortony, ed., *Metaphor and Thought* (Cambridge: Cambridge University Press, 1993); "mental models," as developed by D. Gentner and A. Stevens, eds., *Mental Models* (Mahwah, NJ: Lawrence Erlbaum, 1983); and "idealized cognitive models," as developed by G. Lakoff, *Women, Fire, and Dangerous Things* (Chicago: University of Chicago Press, 1987). However, these alternatives place a stronger emphasis on the cognitive aspects of the processes than intended, and I was seeking to widen how they are viewed by capturing the broader interplay between concept, device, and image.

11. Chaim Perelman is a key writer on the nature of rhetoric, particularly his books C. Perelman, *The New Rhetoric and the Humanities: Essays on Rhetoric and Its Implications* (Dortrecht: D. Reidel, 1979), and *The Realm of Rhetoric* (Notre Dame, IL: University of Notre Dame Press, 1982).

12. See G. Kennedy, *A New History of Classical Rhetoric* (Princeton, NJ: Princeton University Press, 1994).

13. I will stick to the term "devices" or "rhetorical devices" in order to avoid unfamiliar jargon, but the term "trope" is still widely used. For further discussion, see P. Dixon, *Rhetoric* (London: Methuen, 1971).

14. See summaries by E. Winterowd, *Rhetoric: A Synthesis* (New York: Holt, Rinehart & Winstone, 1968) and W. Booth, *The Rhetoric of Rhetoric* (Malden: Blackwell, 2004).

15. Immanuel Kant, *Critique of Judgement* (Oxford: Oxford University Press, 1952, 1892) I, section 53.

16. This decline in the status of rhetoric is described in detail by B. Vickers, *In Defence of Rhetoric* (Oxford: Clarendon Press, 1988) and R. Carpenter, *History as Rhetoric* (Columbia: University of South Carolina Press, 1995).

17. T. De Quincey, *Selected Essays on Rhetoric* (Carbondale: Southern Illinois University Press, 2010, 1897) X81, p. 97.

18. See "new rhetoric," discussed in H. Simons, *Rhetoric in the Human Sciences* (London: Sage, 1989) and in S. Thomas, *What Is the New Rhetoric?* (Newcastle: Cambridge Scholars, 2007).

19. A key work on classifying devices has been the Belgium group of rhetoricians, "Group Mu," in J. Dubois et al., *A General Rhetoric* (Baltimore, MD: Johns Hopkins University Press, 1981, 1970).

20. See examples of these different applications of rhetoric in V. Leymore, *Hidden Myth: Structure and Symbolism in Advertising* (London: Heinemann, 1975); J. Combs and G. Freedman, *Narrative Therapy: The Social Construction of Preferred Realities* (New York: W. W. Norton, 1996); P. Corcoran, *Political Language and Rhetoric* (Brisbane: University of Queensland Press, 1979); and P. Brooks and P. Gewirtz, *Law's Stories: Narrative and Rhetoric in the Law* (New Haven, CT: Yale University Press, 1996).

21. A helpful overview of framing in political communications is provided by D. Chong and J. Druckman in "Framing theory," *Annual Review of Political Science* (10:1, 103–26, 2007), and R. Entman, *Projects of Power: Framing News, Public Opinion, and U.S. Foreign Policy* (Chicago: University of Chicago Press, 2004).

22. See P. Borah, "Conceptual issues in framing theory," *Journal of Communication* (61:2, 246–63, 2011).

23. Of most importance is the holy trinity of devices: metonymy, synecdoche, and metaphor. For discussion, see the collection by R. Dirven and R. Porings, eds., *Metaphor and Metonymy in Comparison and Contrast* (Berlin: Mouton de Gruyter, 2002).

24. W. Gamson & A. Modigliani, "Media discourse and public opinion on nuclear power," *American Journal of Sociology* (95:1, 1–37, 1989).

25. I explore industry rhetoric and framings in *Moral Jeopardy: The Risks of Accepting Money from Tobacco, Alcohol and Gambling Industries* (Cambridge: Cambridge University Press, 2016). See also S. Yoon and T. Lam, "The illusion of righteousness," *BMC Public Health* (13, 630, 2013).

26. The use of rhetoric in religious language is explored in many books, including J. Soskice, *Metaphor and Religious Language* (Oxford: Clarendon Press, 1985); E. MacCormac, *Metaphor and Myth in Science and Religion* (Durham, NC: Duke University Press, 1976); and G. White, *Talking About Spirituality in Health Care Practice* (London: Jessica Kingsley, 2006).

6

Essential Structures

The first enabling frame we will look at, and one Leo has already referenced, approaches death as a key aspect in the structures that enable living and existing to take place. The central idea proposes that since my-death is infrastructural to existence, then regular contact with elements of this infrastructure will bring us into indirect contact with my-death. This discussion will take us right to the edge of what language is capable of expressing, and, for that reason, many of the terms will appear vague and difficult to pin down. However, in a territory concerned with what makes experience possible and, accordingly, what makes language possible, meanings are by their very nature unstable because we can only indirectly hint at what is meant. As stated by Wesley Wildman (2018),

> Our species is obsessed with trying to eff the ineffable—to limn the liminal, to conceive the inconceivable, to speak the unspeakable, to say the unsayable. This obsession shoots colorful threads through the tapestry of human language.[1]

So this is the spirit of what this chapter intends: Is there a way to look at the role of my-death as part of the primordial structures that underpin our existence?

The Structure of Being

Leo's encounter with the inevitability of my-death at Aunty Sue's graveside, followed by his energetic conversations with Stan and Brenda, had prompted an intense interest in the meaning of my-death. It galvanized for him the need to find a way of conceptualizing my-death with which he could feel comfortable and that would provide him with a framework for interacting with my-death in the future.

It was mid-Saturday morning, and Leo had taken a break from his studies to visit Stan. "Over the last few months I've been trying to look up and read some books on death."

"I hope your mother doesn't know," commented Stan.

"Hmm, yes, I make sure she doesn't see what I'm reading. It would just upset her. . . . One book I stumbled across in a bookshop is by an American psychologist, Irving Yalom, called, *Staring at the Sun: Overcoming the Terror of Death*.[2] In it he talks in quite a personal way about his anxiety concerning his own death, and argues that mortality haunts us all our lives."

"Hmm, I'd say he's right there," commented Stan wryly.

"He also draws a lot on other writers; for example, Sigmund Freud."

"I thought Freud wrote mainly about how children have sexual interests in their mothers?"

"Yes, but apparently Freud also wrote a lot about death.[3] Like Yalom, he argues that most people push death to one side and avoid talking about it. . . . And the other guy Yalom keeps quoting was a German philosopher, writing well over 100 years ago, by the name of Friedrich Nietzsche. So I Googled him and found he also talks about the need to embrace death as part of saying 'yes' to life.[4] But, then, his writings led me to another German philosopher, Martin Heidegger, who's written a fair bit about death. And, get this, he was a Nazi!"[5]

"Oh, I have heard him. Isn't he virtually impossible to read?"

"Yeah, that's right. So, I went to the university library and took out his main work, *Being and Time*, and I found, sure enough, I couldn't make head nor tail of it." Leo paused to sip his coffee. "Then I talked to a friend studying philosophy and he suggested reading writers who wrote about Heidegger. I went back to the library and found shelf after shelf of books devoted to him, so then I narrowed my search down to books about his ideas on death. I found two books that were quite helpful, one by David Krell and the other by Carol White."[6]

"Oh great. So Heidegger wrote a couple of books, and another thousand other books are written to explain what he meant," joked Stan. "Okay, tell me what you think he's saying."

"Hmm, well it's complicated," said Leo. "From what I can make out, he's primarily interested in the nature of what he calls 'Being' with a capital 'B,' and the various ways it connects with ordinary things or 'beings' within a small 'b,' you know, beings like houses, cars, planets, dogs, insects, and so forth. One of the central functions of each of these beings is to manifest the essential and unifying power of Being with a capital 'B.'"

"Okay, I'm with you: capital 'B' Being shines through all small 'b' beings."

"Now, what Heidegger does next is rather crafty. He distinguishes us human beings, us experiencing individuals, as what he calls *Dasein*, roughly translated as 'there-being.' See, he thinks of us as located beings, participating in the connection between other beings and this capital 'B' Being."

"Hmm, I'll need to think a little about this maneuver," said Stan, pausing and raising one of his hands to his forehead. "So, as conscious experiencing 'there-beings,' each of us becomes like a torch, or a mirror, shining Being through other beings."

"Yes, kind of . . . that'll do for now," said Leo smiling, a little surprised at how quickly the old man engaged with these difficult ideas. "See, lots of his writings are about the structures that are in place that make it possible for my *Dasein*—or 'there-being'—to do what it does."[7]

Heidegger drew on the ideas of his predecessor and teacher Edmund Husserl, father of phenomenology. Phenomenology aims to examine the essence of a particular experienced object by, first, suspending judgment on the existence of that object; second, by viewing it from several different angles or positions; and, finally, by identifying the essential ingredients of how that object is experienced.[8] This sequence may seem unnecessary for objects like mountains or tables, but it is a powerful approach when looking at more experientially embedded objects such as "home," "injustice," or "loneliness."[9] For example, in exploring the nature of a hallucination, the existence of the perceived object is put to one side in order to concentrate on the details of how it is perceived—it is pink, in the shape of an elephant, and moving toward me.[10] This setting aside of concerns about existence enables a rich description of how objects of consciousness are experienced. Heidegger then applied these methods as a basis for his study of the nature of existence ("fundamental ontology") and related aspects of experience such as "time," "world," and "things."

In pursuing this specialized phenomenology, Heidegger recognized that for Being to manifest itself in surrounding things, there needed to be a situated channel to provide the means by which such manifestation could take place. Cleverly he avoided concepts like consciousness and subjectivity and instead came up with his own term, *Dasein* ("there-being"), in which its

central function in revealing the Being of individual beings is clearly understood. Indeed, he repeatedly emphasized the nature of this central function.

> *Dasein itself . . . gets its ontological understanding of itself in the first instance*
> *from those entities which it itself is not but which it encounters "within" its*
> *world, and from the Being which they possess.*[11]

In this way *Dasein* mediates between Being and beings, and it does so across
the backdrop—or "horizon"—of experienced time. To capture this, he characterized *Dasein* as being "thrown" into experienced time across a threefold
structure made up of "Being ahead of itself" (future), "Being already in"
(past), and "Being alongside" (present).[12]

Stan poured out coffees and opened up a packet of chocolate-coated
cookies. He realized how much he was enjoying this conversation, but he
didn't want his enthusiasm to distract Leo.

Leo resumed his account of Heidegger's ideas. "Now, part of the study
of *Dasein* concerns the nature of how we experience time. I must admit
I hadn't thought about this much, and, in studying physics and chemistry,
I've become so used to presenting time as a line on a graph, which, when you
think about it, captures very little about how we actually experience time."

"Yeah, I can see that. Lines on a graph just reduce time to something in
space, which, of course, misses out many of its other properties, like how we
can't really see into the future."[13]

"Exactly, and, as Heidegger points out, we travel through our individual
bubbles of time in quite a structured way; for instance, we occupy the present with our past flowing out behind us and our future is approaching,
full of uncertain possibilities. This happens all through our time on this
planet, and it structures everything in our experience including thoughts,
emotions, and intuitions. He gives this structure a funny name, the 'ecstatic
unity of temporality.'"[14]

"Goodness, that's a mouthful."

"That's nothing; you should try to deal with the rest of the strange terms
he comes up with," Leo smiled and dunked a cookie in his coffee, then licked
the melted chocolate. "Any rate, there's one aspect of the structure of temporality to which he pays particular attention and that concerns *Dasein*'s
relationship to death. He calls this 'being toward death'—although some
writers prefer to talk about it as 'being toward the end.' What I think he

means by this is that as long as I, as *Dasein*, am around, I face forward to this possibility, the possibility that I no longer exist; well, actually, he called it an impossible possibility, but that's another story.[15] See, my death stands there before me, whether I see it or not; it stands there and constantly underpins and defines for me what it means to exist."

"Hmm, I think I've got a vague sense of what he means. So, death is integral to our experience of time, and, in some ways, death is one of the organizing principles for time."

Leo nodded thoughtfully. "Yes, I cannot think of life without death. As I said before, a life without death is a nonsense; one is predicated on the other. What's more, you can't think it because it belongs to the basic structure that enables existence to take place, including the way I think and the way I speak. I mean, just as you can't think time or space, but you know them intimately because they are conditions that make daily experience possible, it's the same thing with death; it is integral and intrinsic to what it means to be alive."

In line with points we have discussed in previous chapters, Heidegger was primarily interested in my-death rather than death in general, and he approached it as an event in life, "As death comes, it vanishes. Mortals die death in life. In death mortals become im-mortal."[16] By speaking about being "im-mortal" Heidegger was not suggesting *Dasein* continues in some form of immortal afterlife; rather, he was pointing to the unknowable nature of death as an endpoint in experienced time.

> The "ending" which we have in view when we speak of death, does not signify *Dasein's Being-at-the-end, but a Being-toward-the-end of this entity. Death is a way to be, which Dasein takes over as soon as it is.*[17]

As *Dasein* looks out into the future across the horizon of time, the inevitability of an endpoint presents itself. My-death, as this inevitable endpoint, does not present itself as an auxiliary or optional part of time; rather it appears as a core part of time's role in the very structuring of Being.

> As long as Dasein is, something is always still outstanding: what it can be and will be. But the "end" itself belongs to what is outstanding. The "end" of being-in-the-world is death. This end, belonging to the potentiality-of-being, that is, to existence, limits and defines the possible totality of Dasein.[18]

What follows from accepting my-death as a necessary structural element in the nature of existence (this being-toward-death) repositions it as an integral part of what it means to exist.[19] So, in a way, if you know about and embrace life, then you know about and embrace death; they co-actualize each other.[20]

Another angle Heidegger took with my-death was to characterize it as a "Nothing" or "nothingness" or a location for "the mystery of Being itself." This further reinforced the unknowable and unspeakable nature of my-death not as an empty hole with nothing to reveal, but rather as a point of invisibility because it is embedded as a necessary part of the fundamental structures of Being.

> *Death is the shrine of Nothing, that is, of that which in every respect is never merely something that merely exists, but which nevertheless presences even as the mystery of Being itself. As the shrine of Nothing, death harbors within itself the presencing of Being. As the shrine of Nothing, death is the shelter of Being. We now call mortals mortals—not because their earthly life comes to an end, but because they are capable of death as death. Mortals are who they are, as mortals, present in the shelter of Being. They are the presencing relation to Being as Being.[21]*

As proposed in Chapter 3, the inevitability of my-death is both unknowable and unspeakable, a "Nothing" as Heidegger calls it, but, according to him, because it resides in what is inherent to the very structure, the very givenness, of life, it is to some extent revealed, and revealed enough to enable some form of connection, if not with the mind, a connection in some other fundamental way.

Finitude

Finitude is an important concept when talking about personal mortality. It is used by a number of thinkers as a catch-all concept that refers to a vast variety of ways in which we are aware of the boundaries or limits that constrain our everyday existence.[22] Heidegger employed the concept throughout his thinking to characterize the full extent of individual human boundedness and its relationship to my-death.[23] He even described finitude as "the constant, though generally concealed, shudder that pervades all existence."[24]

On Sunday afternoon, the following day, Leo let himself in through Stan's back door and found him dozing in his armchair with the book on death he had borrowed from Brenda splayed open on his lap.

"Oh, oh . . . Leo . . . ," Stan struggled to sit upright and focus his eyes on his visitor. "Was I sleeping?"

"Only snoozing." Leo sat down on the couch opposite Stan and leaned forward with an enthusiastic smile. "Look, I've read a bit more about Heidegger and death, and I want to talk it through."

Stan's mind had all but emerged from its fog. He recalled how much he had enjoyed their conversation yesterday, so he was keen for Leo to continue. "Okay, good . . . give it a whirl."

"Hmm, another concept that Heidegger keeps using in relation to death is 'finitude.' He wrote about it in several of his books, two of which I looked up.[25] I didn't know what it meant at first, but I'm gradually getting a sense of it."

"Hmm, 'finitude,'" commented Stan. "Do you mean something to do with the way we are finite?"

"Yes, that's it. It refers to all the limitations and constraints that hold each of us together as individual existing entities. There are lots of ways in which this happens."

"Okay, like what?"

"Well, at this very moment, my presence here is constrained by time. It's nine in the morning on Sunday the eighth of September, 2019. This is today. I occupy no other day; yesterday has become inaccessible and tomorrow has yet to come."

"Hmm, but that's just the nature of things."

"Exactly: the ways in which my being is constrained belong to the nature of things. That's what I'm saying," said Leo laughing and rocking backward on the couch. "And, what's more, I'm constrained by place. I'm here and not there; at this moment I can't be anywhere else. In a few moments I could be over there, but then I'd be no longer here. I'm always here. And I can't walk through that wall over there; I have to go through the door. I'm constantly constrained by solid boundaries."

"What about time travel? That delivers you to a different time and place, and often in movies time travelers go back to meet their younger selves."

"Ah, but that's never happened; it's a fiction; an amusing fiction, but really impossible. See, even in time travel you're stuck in a singular situation; you carry it around with you."

"Hmm, wouldn't it be great to be in several places at once," mused Stan.

"Yes, that would be nice, but it would require disrupting the structures that hold us together. And there's another part of this structure: I'm always constrained by my body; it constantly holds me in place. My skin is this fleshy container that wraps around the blood, bone, organs, and fluids that keep me alive. At no time am I free from my body, and through it I derive all my senses, all my thoughts, and all my emotions; these constantly collide into patterns in my consciousness. They continuously condition what I'm experiencing."

For Heidegger, these aspects of what it means to be finite and finitude itself is not merely an aspect of what it means to exist, but a vital part of making our existence possible.

> *Finitude is not some property that is merely attached to us, but is our funda-*
> *mental way of being. If we wish to become what we are, we cannot abandon*
> *this finitude or deceive ourselves about it, but must safeguard it. Such pres-*
> *ervation is the innermost process of our being finite, i.e., it is our innermost*
> *becoming finite. Finitude only is in truly becoming finite.*[26]

This extends the reach of my-death into a much wider arena than a focused endpoint. In this way my-death becomes linked to the everyday aspects of our limited existence.[27]

"But," continued Leo energetically, "I'm not only constrained by my physical situation, I'm also constrained by who I am as a person. I am constantly jostled by fears, hopes, and preferences, and these lead me to think and act in particular ways—particular ways and not in other ways."

"Okay, that's right to some extent," said Stan.

"Like, you know, my Mom . . . she frets a lot about different things, and as you've told me before, she's a worrier; this is her personality. And you can't really expect her to be otherwise; she'll never approach situations, like some people do, totally relaxed and not worried about outcomes."

"But she could change; anyone can change. She could take up meditation, or exercise more, or go to a therapist; these would all make her less worried."

"Yes, she could do that, and it is true that the limits of my personality are never totally fixed; but they are fixed to some extent. I think I'm a bit of a risk-taker; always on the lookout for new adventures. I could work at calming that down, but I know as soon as I spot the prospect for a new spree, I'm off. It's in my nature."

"I suppose you're right," said Stan thoughtfully. "When I look back over the span of my lifetime, at my friends and myself, the combination of genetics, upbringing, and life-experiences seems to coalesce into a potent mix which seems to hold each of us together as individuals. I notice that whenever I meet people from my younger years, like at a school reunion, it always surprises me how little they've changed, despite it being fifty or more years since we met."

"Added to this, I am continually constrained by the way I see things; by the implicit biases and beliefs handed down to me from Mom, my friends, and the media around me. I am fated at each moment to look out at things from a particular angle, from a particular vantage point, full of all the influences and prejudices that belong to being a twenty-one-year-old white male."

"Hmm, I get it; I'm just as much a product of my time and influences as you."

"So you see why Heidegger developed this concept of finitude; these constraining processes all acting together to hold me in place."

"So where does death come in?"

"Well, I'm still trying to sort that out. Look, I've only been reading Heidegger's ideas for a few months, and I know there is much more to learn. I guess, at this stage, the main thing is he's helped me appreciate how death contributes to the fundamental structuring of what it means for me to be alive, and I think death has an important relationship to finitude. I'm by no means on top of what he's hammering on about, but I've read enough to know he's onto something."

Indeed Heidegger does continually connect my-death to the broader array of constraints that comprise personal finitude. He took a particular interest in finitude's relationship to the bounds of what we both know and what we can say.[28] But he also repeatedly emphasized the pivotal role finitude plays in the fundamental structuring elements of time and vital connections with manifestations of Being. For example in an all-encompassing footnote he stated:

Existence as a mode of being is in itself finitude and as such it is possible only on the ground of the understanding of Being. . . . On the ground of the

understanding of Being man is the "there"; due to this being the there the
opening break toward the world occurs, so that the world and its entities
as such can be given to a self. More primordial than man is the finitude of
Dasein within him. . . . [W]e do not need to ask toward a relation of the un-
derstanding of Being to the finitude in the human being. It is itself the inner-
most essence of finitude.[29]

This is a difficult passage to decipher, but what is clear is the way Heidegger was positioning finitude as a central link between individual there-being (*Dasein*) and Being as a whole. What attracted Leo to these ideas was the way in which my-death and finitude connect and their role in the essential structures for Being as it manifests itself in the affairs of everyday life.

My-Death Is Intrinsic

Scholars tackling Heidegger's understanding of death, such as Joachim Oberst (2009) and David Krell (1986), have highlighted the intrinsic connections between Being, finitude, and my-death. Leo's young and inquisitive mind had eagerly grasped some of what was intended, but he now sought to take these ideas further and apply them to his immediate circumstances.

While Leo recognized the unthinkableness of my-death, he also realized how it somehow still managed to assert its presence. He felt drawn to find ways of sharing his ideas with others in the hope of exploring what it meant in life. He wondered whether the person closest to him, his mother, might be interested in talking it over.

Leo and Mandy were sitting at the kitchen table catching up before preparing dinner. Leo looked directly across at Mandy. "Mom, have you ever noticed how everything in your life feels constrained?"

"Hmm, yes, constrained. . . ." Mandy was adapting to the switch in topic. "I don't really like having to get up every morning and work in the shop. It's the last thing I want to do; but I need to, otherwise we wouldn't have any food, or a house to live in."

"Yes, I know such things can be annoying, but constraints like that help configure your life. It's like . . . it's like the friction that gives life some form of traction."

"You might look at it that way, but it's also a damn nuisance. Often I dream of being beamed out and beyond my daily grind; to escape the financial hassles, the traffic, the housework . . . and the cold and miserable loneliness I sometimes feel."

"Hmm, but don't you think these limitations also have a positive side?"

"Positive? What's positive about endless worry?"

"Well, I just think that without constraints and limitations, life would disappear into a meaningless void. You imagine it. Without limits we could do anything, be anything, go anywhere . . . but then, what would be the point? If you can do anything you like, then what you do manage to do is hardly any form of achievement."

"I'm not so sure," said Mandy. "In each moment, with each achievement . . . I would be happy with that in itself."

"Yeah, but imagine if you went on living; on and on, living a life without end. You could then climb the tallest mountain, write the best novel, graduate as a doctor, then as a lawyer, then become a professor. . . . You would just keep on going and going in an endless sequence. And eventually anything that stands in your way could be overcome; it's just a matter of time." Leo paused and glanced at the baffled look on Mandy's face "And that's another thing, if time carries on and on then it, too, would turn into a featureless blur."

"But, that could happen. I don't think the constraints of life are what give it meaning."

"Well, you just imagine living a life without death. Everything would become possible over time, but after a while it would all merge into one. It would all become one amorphous, meaningless blob."

Mandy looked uncomfortable. "I think it is possible to think of a life beyond death."

"The fact of my future death is core to what makes me finite. It belongs to what structures how I exist."

"Ah, so all this is leading to talk of death," said Mandy, now frowning at Leo across the table.

Leo cast a defiant stare back. "Yes, it's about death."

"Look, I told you before," she said with her voice harsh and shrill. "You need to stop going on and on about death. It's doing no good." She raised her right hand and pointed at him. "No, Leo, I'm sick of it. Just stop!" She stood up and continued in a low trembling voice. "I've worked so hard all these years to give you a good start in life, and now all you talk about is death. Please, please . . . just stop it."

Leo was attempting to present finitude and its association with my-death as integral to what enables life to garner value and meaning. He felt sure that assumptions of endless happiness and a continuing afterlife entailed conceal-ment of the reality of my-death and, in the process, involved turning away from a stronger and perhaps more authentic understanding of the human condition. Moreover, for him, this realization was not like other forms of learning where, once a discovery is made, it is stored away in order to ad-vance other learning. He felt the urge to continue building this idea into a stronger awareness.

Following in the footsteps of Heidegger, the Russian-born French thinker Alexandre Kojève said of this awareness,

> *Since Man is born from finitude, it is only by thinking of death and by speaking of it that he is truly what he is: discourse conscious of itself and of its origin. . . .*
>
> *. . . Now it is only in becoming conscious of his finitude, and therefore of his death, that a man truly becomes conscious of himself. For he is finite and mortal.*[30]

But who could Leo speak with? Who would help him traverse this un-stable territory through to a solid and ongoing awareness? He sensed the relationships here were complex, more complex than they seemed, and he recognized he needed assistance in navigating the subtle distinctions and complex interactions between the various facets of both finitude and my-death.

It was early evening when Brenda walked into the living room to find Leo sitting in semi-darkness staring at the wall. "Leo, you're very quiet."

At first he did not respond. As Brenda motioned to leave, he declared, "I just had an argument with Mom."

Brenda walked across and turned on the lamp in the corner of the room. "What on earth about? You normally get on so well."

"Oh, the usual. She hates me talking about anything to do with death. She just cuts me down; then I feel so pissed off she won't share this with me."

Brenda sat down in the armchair opposite.

Leo turned and stared directly at her. "Brenda, how do you feel about being limited and constrained all the time? I mean, I'm stuck here in this place, this mundane place . . . stuck in my body, stuck in this personality, stuck in this mind looking out at an overly familiar world."

These seemed to Brenda alarming statements; such negative views. She wondered if he was depressed, or worse, whether he was thinking about suicide again. Perhaps she should probe him for more detail. "You seem to worry a lot about such things."

"No, it doesn't bother me," he replied glancing back at her with a perplexed expression. "On the contrary, I see them as vital to the structuring of my life."

"Oh, good," she sighed. "To answer your question, I guess I find constraints difficult: you know, having to go to work every day . . . and to observe signs of my body's approaching aging. Sometimes I hate these things, and it makes me want to break out of being right here, right now; to travel by a magic carpet to an exotic land, to jump into a time machine into the future."

"Hmm, but I reckon these boundaries and limitations are good; they are part of the overriding framework that holds us together as existing individuals, and therefore we should embrace them rather than try to overcome them or ignore them."

"Okay, I can see how, in general, you might view them as necessary. But, at the time, when they're bothering me, I do sometimes really, really want to break free."

"What's more, I see these boundaries as connected to death."

"Oh death again. You know your. . . ."

" . . . no, no, listen to me," he interrupted. "I need to talk to someone about it otherwise I'll explode." He smiled faintly as he observed her nod. "I think of my own death as an ultimate constraint, like a super-boundary powering other limitations that surround me. Other things that hold me, such as my containment in time and containment in my body, are beholden to the overarching power of death."

"I'm not sure I quite get what you're saying."

"Look, you think about it. Death is embedded in every boundary; it sits behind as the powerhouse that drives every constraint." He glanced across at Brenda's bemused expression and tried to think of other ways to convince her. "Take time, for instance. Time can be interpreted as how long you feel you have to live; after all, that's the only time that really matters.

And your position in space is framed by solid barriers, walls and buildings; you'd be severely injured if you tried to run through them. Death also stands there behind the walls stopping you."

"Yes, that's true, the possibility of me dying does ultimately constrain me. I see every day at work how thin the membrane is that separates life from death."

"As for the frailty and vulnerability of your body, each bodily deterioration—when you go bald, develop wrinkles, lose fertility, become less strong and flexible—each of these have special meaning because of their relationship to your approaching death. But, more than that, they are actually playing a solid part in your ultimate fate."

"Oh, Leo," sighed Brenda, "I must say you are painting quite a bleak picture. I'm not sure I can see death as spread so widely through everything."

"Can't you see what I'm saying? Death is a vital part of the structures that drive us. It's integral to life because it comprises the girders set into the walls that constrain and frame each moment of our existence."

Leo used the metaphor of a building structure to convey the idea of my-death providing the inner strength for all the boundaries that contribute to personal finitude; and, in return, our constant contact with these boundaries enables us to maintain some indirect contact with my-death. While my-death remains unspeakable, its role in bolstering the solidity of the multitudinous boundaries of personal finitude brings it partially out of the shadows and provides a basis for some form of engagement. The German-American theologian Paul Tillich said it this way:

> *The fact that man never is satisfied with any stage of his finite development, the fact that nothing finite can hold him, although finitude is his destiny, indicates the indissoluble relation of everything finite to being-itself. Being-itself is not infinity: it is that which lies beyond the polarity of finitude and infinite self-transcendence. Being-itself manifests itself to finite being in the infinite drive of the finite beyond itself.*[31]

Tillich, like Heidegger, saw finitude as situated at the core of what it means to be human and since we can connect with finitude on a daily basis, through its representations in what bounds and constrains us, this enables us to find indirect ways of linking up with my-death.

Leo burst through the back door into Stan's kitchen where he was standing at the sink washing his dishes.

"Goodness," exclaimed Stan holding his breath. "You did give me half a fright."

Leo strode purposively over to the table and sat watching Stan wiping down his counter. "I tried talking this stuff over with both Mom and Brenda, but neither of them are on the same wavelength."

Stan could see his disappointment. "Okay, tell me where you've got to."

Leo ran through his ideas of death as the powerhouse for driving the meaning of other boundaries and limitations.

When he had finished, Stan smiled at him and commented, "So you're arguing death is like a super-boundary, a meta-limit; like all aspects of finitude owe their force to the link they have with death?"

"Yes, and because I see finitude as contributing positively to the structure of life, all I'm trying to do is find a way of staying connected with it. . . . Is that too much to ask?"

"Not too much . . . but, tell me how this helps you connect with death?"

"Ah, that's easy," replied Leo with a smile spreading across his face. "If the fact of my death is the powerhouse of finitude, and finitude in its many forms is what structures my existence, then whenever I embrace my existence, I'm also embracing finitude, and, accordingly, I am indirectly embracing my own death. It's a linkage line: me-existence-finitude-death and death-finitude-existence-me, all wired up and vitalizing each other."

"So, you see death as intrinsic to life, as a necessary condition for what it means to exist, and you recognize that because of your positive embrace of finitude?"

"Yes, that's right. And now I reckon my challenge is to find ways to hold this in my mind so it grows stronger and forms into a constant awareness." Leo stared earnestly at Stan. "At this stage it's only a weak connection, one easily washed away. I want it to strengthen to a point that I feel constantly connected with death."

Leo had made use of Heidegger's thinking to configure in his mind the idea of essential structures as a frame that enabled him to set up an ongoing relationship with my-death. He achieved this by means of four interlocking realizations. First, he rejected the notion of life after death on the basis that it was a category mistake—and, perhaps a contradiction in terms. The idea of an afterlife involves abstracting life away from my-death; it involves putting my-death to one side and imagining life as continuing on forever. But when death is viewed as a necessary condition for what it means to exist, such abstraction is no longer possible. Second, he saw the prospect of his own death, as distinct from the death of others, as standing resolutely before him as an inevitable and unavoidable endpoint to his existence. This endpoint profoundly challenged the whole of existence and, as such, alerted him to the intrinsic part my-death plays in the structuring of time and in the presencing of Being. Third, he saw my-death as having a structural function in powering the many boundaries and limitations that surround each of us and define who we are. These he understood collectively as "finitude" and as composed of the diverse range of limitations that constantly surround us, including those associated with time, place, body, person, and perspective. Finitude differs from my-death in that it is constantly and visibly active in daily life; it shapes and organizes everyday experience and provides the substance for individual identity. Fourth, he recognized how at the tail-end of each of the boundaries that comprise personal finitude lurks the potency of my-death. He visualized my-death as an ultimate constraint or meta-boundary that provides the motive force for all that limits and constrains each of us. For him it followed, accordingly, that by accessing finitude, by paying attention to the boundaries and constraints that surround him, he would then be indirectly connecting to my-death and that this, over time, could form into a solid and ongoing awareness.

Leo's use of the enabling frame of essential structures will, from now on, provide the basis for how he thinks and how he talks to the other characters about my-death. But there are three further alternative frames to consider.

Notes

1. W. J. Wildman, *Effing the Ineffable: Existential Mumblings at the Limits of Language* (Albany: State University of New York Press, 2018) p. ix.
2. Irvin Yalom, *Staring at the Sun: Overcoming the Terror of Death* (San Francisco: Jossey-Bass, 2010), also published as an article, "Staring at the sun," *Humanistic Psychologist* (36:3–4, 283–97, 2008).
3. Freud wrote two key essays on death: "Timely thoughts on war and death" and "Our relation to death" in *Reflections on War and Death* (New York: Moffat, Yard & Co., 1918) and discussed by L. Razinsky, *Freud, Psychoanalysis and Death* (Cambridge: Cambridge University Press, 2013).

4. Yalom's fascination with Nietzsche's ideas inspired him to pen a fictional account of Nietzsche in psychotherapy, *When Nietzsche Wept: A Novel of Obsession* (New York: Basic Books, 1992).

5. Heidegger's membership and active involvement with the Nazi Party from April 1933 to February 1934 has been very controversial, with some arguing that his thinking aligns with basic Nazi ideas and others saying that he was only temporarily involved and that his thinking was separate from his politics. For discussion of the former, see H. D. Sluga, *Heidegger's Crisis: Philosophy and Politics in Nazi Germany* (Cambridge, MA: Harvard University Press, 1995).

6. Key commentaries on Heidegger and death include David Krell, *Intimations of Mortality: Time, Truth, and Finitude in Heidegger's Thinking of Being* (University Park: Pennsylvania State University Press, 1986); Carol White, *Time and Death: Heidegger's Analysis of Finitude* (Aldershot: Ashgate, 2005); Joachim Oberst, *Heidegger on Language and Death* (London: Continuum, 2009); and George Pattison, *Heidegger on Death* (Surrey: Ashgate, 2013).

7. Hedegger's work is vast, spanning six decades of writing. This chapter touches on only a small sample of his contribution to the history of ideas, and descriptions of his conceptualization of death in terms of essential structures is a simplification of the many different angles he took on Being and death.

8. Husserl describes these procedures in more detail in *Cartesian Meditations: An Introduction to Phenomenology* (Dordrecht: Kluwer Academic, 1999).

9. A considerable amount has been written about phenomenological research methods. See C. Moustakas, *Phenomenological Research Methods* (Thousand Oaks, CA: Sage, 1994).

10. Husserl referred to this setting aside of judgment on the existence of objects as "epoché," and this process of systematic reduction forms an important part of phenomenological research methods.

11. Martin Heidegger, *Being and Time* (Oxford: Basil Blackwell, 1973) p. 85 (author's emphasis removed, here and in subsequent quotes).

12. David Krell describes this threefold structure in this way in *Intimations of Mortality*, p. 54.

13. The French philosopher Henri Bergson also championed a critique of the spatialization of time in *Time and Free Will* (New York: Macmillan, 1910).

14. Carol White talks about this as "the ecstases of timeliness" in *Time and Death*, p. 96.

15. Jacques Derrida criticizes Heidegger's formulation of death as both possible and impossible by claiming it relies on viewing death as a boundary. He offers an alternative formulation with his term *Aporia*, which he talks of as a "non-passable situation," in *Aporias* (Stanford, CA: Stanford University Press, 1993). Havi Carel in "Temporal finitude and finitude of possibility," *International Journal of Philosophical Studies* (15:4 541–56, 2007), points out how critics have confused Heidegger's notion of death with something to do with the event that ends life, when he is really talking about death "both as temporal finitude and as finitude of possibility," p. 541.

16. Quoted in J. Oberst, *Heidegger on Language and Death*, p. 31, and originally from Heidegger's *Holderlins Erde und Himmel* (1959).

17. M. Heidegger, *Being and Time*, p. 289.

18. Ibid., pp. 233–34.

19. Heidegger refers to *Dasein*'s potentiality for a relationship to my-death as "authenticity" and contrasts it with the inauthentic evasion of death as discussed in Chapter 4. This understanding of authenticity is explored in detail by Carol White in *Time and Death*, particularly chapters 1 and 3.

20. This is a simplification of Heidegger's detailed analysis of death and is summarized more thoroughly by Sean Ireton in *An Ontological Study of Death* (Pittsburgh, PA: Duquesne University Press, 2007) pp. 229–80.

21. M. Heidegger, "The thing," in *Poetry, Language, Thought* (New York: Harper & Row, 1971) p. 176.

22. Writers on finitude include followers of Heidegger, such as Jacques Taminiaux, *Dialectic and Difference: Finitude in Modern Thought* (New York: Humanities Press, 1985) and Alejandro Vallega, *Sense and Finitude* (Albany: State University of New York Press, 2009), as well as independent thinkers such as Paul Ricoeur, *Fallible Man* (New York: Fordham University Press, 1986), and Francesco Adorno, "Against posthuman ideology: Aesthetics and finitude of the individual," *Res: Anthropology and Aesthetics* (57/58, 344–54, 2010).

23. Heidegger's ideas on finitude and boundedness are presented in *The Fundamental Concepts of Metaphysics: World, Finitude, Solitude* (Bloomington: Indiana University Press, 1995).

24. Quoted by C. White, *Time and Death*, p. 21.

25. Heidegger's early writing on finitude can be found mostly in Heidegger, *Being and Time* and *Kant and the Problem of Metaphysics* (Bloomington: Indiana University Press, 1997).

26. M. Heidegger from *Fundamental Concepts of Metaphysics*, p. 6.

27. Oren Magid, in "Heidegger on human finitude," *European Journal of Philosophy* (25:3, 440–62, 2017), argues that, according to Heidegger's concept of finitude, "the intelligibility of ourselves, the world, and everything within the world is grounded or anchored in a final end" (p. 660).

28. In Heidegger's book on Immanuel Kant's philosophy, *Kant and the Problem of Metaphysics*, he looks in depth at the bounds of knowledge. In later work, he focused more on finitude and language, particularly in *The Fundamental Concepts of Metaphysics*. Detailed analysis is provided by J. Oberst in *Heidegger on Language and Death* and by C. White in *Time and Death*, particularly chapter 5.

29. M. Heidegger in *Kant and the Problem of Metaphysics*, p. 228f.

30. Alexandre Kojève, "The idea of death in the philosophy of Hegel," in D. Keenan, ed., *Hegel and Contemporary Continental Philosophy* (Albany: State University of New York Press, 2004) p. 45. With influences from both Heidegger and Marx, Kojève provided a new analysis of Hegel's philosophy, and this quote comes from this analysis.

31. Paul Tillich, *Systematic Theology* (London: Nisbet & Co., 1953) p. 191.

7

Passionate Suffusion

The second enabling frame, passionate suffusion, focuses on pursuing a relationship to my-death in the form of a more intensely personal engagement. It is, in some ways, consistent with the essential structures frame in viewing my-death as an integral part of all existence, but it develops this into a more concentrated involvement by treating it less as a conceptual relationship and more as a relationship of passion in which the presence of my-death radiates with dynamic energy through all things. But before discussing this further, something happened to Stan which triggered a reappraisal of his relationship to my-death.

Stan enjoyed starting his day with a cooked breakfast. It was an important routine; it set up the rhythm for the remainder of his day. He placed bread into the toaster, heated a pan and put on a pot of water to boil. Into the pan he placed two small sausages, a rasher of bacon, then sliced in a few mushrooms. When the water was boiling, he carefully broke in two eggs.

All this while, his various conversations with Brenda and Leo were running through his head. Leo seems so confident about the finality of death and remarkably relaxed about its consequences. Perhaps it's something to do with his age. Brenda, on the other hand, seems to have a more sophisticated, more nuanced understanding, but it's unclear what she actually believes about death.

He turned the stove off and scraped the sausages, bacon, and mushrooms onto the toast. What this needed was some ketchup. He took the bottle out of the fridge and tried to unscrew it, but the top had dried up and seized. He placed a tea-towel over the bottle cap to increase his grip and twisted harder . . . then harder.

Without warning, a pain shot through the upper left side of his body focusing at a point just below his shoulder. This was quickly followed by powerful aching in his chest.

He sat down in the chair, panting. Something's going wrong . . . but it'll pass . . . I don't need anyone's help. Perhaps I'll feel better with something to eat.

He turned in his chair to face his plate, but the pain was getting worse. His chest felt as though it was being squeezed into itself. He panted for more breath. Winston trotted over to lick his hands; the dog seemed to know something wasn't quite right.

He found it increasingly difficult to draw breath, and, by this stage, he knew he needed urgent attention. A surge of fear radiated across his body. This could be it; this could be the end of everything. He tried to stand, but dizziness overtook him and he fell to the floor with the plate and its contents crashing around him.

For Stan, this unexpected moment would act as a circuit-breaker in terms of how he engaged with both his life and his death. Suddenly his lived assumption of continuity had, like a rug, been pulled away from under him. And this was far more than a conceptual realization.

Leo marched into the kitchen and sidled up to where Mandy was mixing the ingredients for a cake.

"Mom, Winston keeps on barking and barking. He's been at it for the last hour. Has Stan gone away?"

"No, I don't think so. He would have said something." She stopped her mixing, gazed out the window, and pondered possibilities. Stan is usually pottering in his garden by now. Why isn't he around? He might've slept in . . . no he never does that. Maybe he's busy with things inside . . . but that doesn't explain Winston's barking.

A scary feeling spread across the base of her stomach. No, something bad has happened.

She marched quickly over and knocked on Stan's door. She pulled urgently on the door handle but found it was firmly locked. "Damn." She placed her ear against the door and could just make out a groan in between Winston's barks. The scary feeling spread from her stomach into her chest. She rushed back into her kitchen.

"Leo, Leo, quick, I need to call an ambulance." Mandy was talking in fast bursts. "Stan is in some kind of trouble." She started dialing the emergency number. "Maybe he's fallen over and knocked his head." She waited impatiently for the ring tone. "Can you try to find some way of getting into his house?"

"Okay," said Leo, jumping up from eating his toast. "Maybe I'll try to force the door open."

Leo threw caution to the wind and, by wedging in a large screwdriver close to the lock, he was able to force the kitchen door open. He entered the kitchen with his heart pounding. "Where's Stan?" As he walked around the counter he nearly tripped over Stan lying splayed on the floor with the oily mess of his breakfast smeared over his shirt. "Oh, Stan, what's happened?"

Stan mumbled a few incoherent words before fading into a groaning oblivion.

Mandy strode in clutching a blanket and an overnight bag, "The ambulance is on its way." She glanced down with a look of dismay at Stan, "Oh, my God, he doesn't look good."

Stan's medical crisis fell like a hammer on a pane of glass, shattering the world around and upsetting his carefully organized routines. Furthermore, as we shall see, a close call with death can have a disruptive impact not only for the person experiencing it but also for those loved ones who are observing what's going on.

Finitude Revisited

Another way of approaching finitude is to see it less as a structural element that manages to keep manifesting itself through all aspects of our finite being and more as a force that dynamically expresses and re-expresses itself in every moment, pulsating as a whole through everything. In this way finitude moves from being seen as a static subterranean element to being experienced in the form of a more immediate and dynamic process. It is thereby promoted from a mechanism by which other forces become manifest to a primordial force in its own right. This is the central idea for this frame; it de-emphasizes my-death as integral to the structures of existence and focuses more on it as a direct and meaningful relationship.

After dinner, the day staff departed the ward, the lights were turned down, and Stan was left lying motionless in semi-darkness. Whereas during the day the ward had been filled with the busy clatter of staff completing forms, dressing wounds, attending to toileting, and organizing feeding, now quietness settled over the beds, interrupted only occasionally by a patient coughing or the stealthy tread of the night nurse.

His mind churned through the events of the past forty-eight hours. Three days ago, at this very time, he'd been living his normal life, confident in the predictability of his routines. Then, without warning, it had all changed. He recalled the panic he experienced during breakfast and the desperation he felt on his way to the hospital. Then the surgeon rushed in to say he needed a heart operation. This prompted a sense of dread to sweep overwhelmingly across his semi-consciousness mind; how fast things can change.

His thoughts drifted onto his recent conversations with Leo and Brenda, particularly those with Leo. For a young person, he seemed so self-assured about death. How can he be so certain? He is undoubtedly correct on one point: death is integral to daily existence; without it, life would turn into an endless meaninglessness. But how can he be so sure it all leads to final annihilation?

Lying there alone in his hospital bed, he felt totally vulnerable. His heart attack had taken him right to the edge of his existence, and he had stared into the abyss. Death was now all around him. He could see death in the various wires and tubes attached to his body: in the heart monitor wire attached to his finger, in the intravenous line plugged in just above his wrist, in the oxygen tubes they sometimes strapped over his nose, in the catheter attached to his penis. Each tube had its function, but their termination on his body signaled his body's mortality.

Death was also playing out with the people who surrounded him. The doctors, nurses, and specialists were continually busy in their important work of preventing patients from dying. They worked in unison to keep death at bay, and the flow of their energy pointed to the continuing presence of death. And, despite their best efforts, it seemed they were just delaying the inevitable; death would ultimately triumph over their craft.

During the afternoon, the heart monitor of an older man in the same room began loudly beeping. Staff ran in with a trolley and attempted to shock him back into life. After three attempts, they wheeled him quickly out. But he didn't return. His bed remained ominously unoccupied.

So, he could see death and finitude dancing all around; the staff were constantly dancing with it, his fellow patients were dancing with it, the machines and wires and tubes were pumping a constant rhythm; even the place itself—the room, the ward, the hospital—seemed to be part of this performance. Death permeated everything. Lying there in the still quiet of the night he could sense it as a palpable presence. He could feel it there like never before; it seemed as though he could reach out and touch it.

His old familiar relationship with death was shifting . . . shifting in a way that was both unnerving and exciting at the same time.

In my book *Navigating Everyday Life: Exploring the Tension between Finitude and Transcendence,*[1] I examine the myriad of ways in which we encounter what bounds and constrains us as we go about our lives. The nature of these boundaries is signaled in momentary flashes that pass us at varying speeds and at varying intensities. Sometimes we barely notice these moments: a fleeting, unnerving shiver down the spine, a nonspecific sense of unease or a momentary worry about the future. In mundane everyday situations, finitude tends to present itself as a vague awareness as we knock up against the bounded nature of our bodies, our minds, and our personal attributes. At other times finitude is encountered in earth-shattering realizations that can shift our whole outlook on life, as occurs during near-death experiences or major traffic accidents. Stan's heart attack was just such an occasion. It brought him undeniably close to my-death and in such a way that he could see my-death as present in the constant action of finitude.

Stan might have achieved this awareness of finitude earlier in his life. The small intimations of finitude can accumulate into something more potent and lead to an experiential, almost visceral awareness that signals a stronger sense of boundedness which extends beyond any specific limitation. This general awareness, in turn, can be signaled and countersignaled in symbolically meaningful moments, such as when he retired or when he first noticed his strength and stamina declining with age. Nonetheless, for various reasons, he had let this awareness slip by; perhaps he was too busy with other matters, or perhaps the passing signals of finitude were too weak, or perhaps a niggling fear of death had prompted him to ignore them. Whatever the reason, it was not until he was directly confronted with his mortality that his mind opened up to the vital power and energy of finitude as it suffuses itself through all parts of his being.[2]

Stan's switch in orientation away from a conceptual understanding toward a passionate embrace of finitude—the enabling frame of passionate suffusion—repositioned my-death as part of a broader process.

Mandy found Stan lying flat out in a hospital bed staring vacantly up at the ceiling. He seemed to have aged significantly since three days before. His cheeks were deflated and slightly grayish, and his unshaven face looked more wrinkled.

Stan's blank expression lit up as he recognized his visitor. "Ah, Mandy, I'm so pleased to see you."

She searched out a vase for the flowers and handed him a get well card. "This is from all of us next door."

"Mandy, you know what?" he said as he opened up the card. "Nice." He looked up at her and smiled. "You know you saved my life. The doctors said if you hadn't come and called the ambulance when you did then I wouldn't be here today. I was right on the edge. It was that close!"

"I'm so glad I did, and you're still here. But I think you really need to thank Winston. It was his barking that raised the alarm."

"Okay, but I'm truly grateful. . . . Thank you."

Mandy stared out the window and, following an awkward pause, asked, "So, what have you been up to while you're in here?"

"Ah, there's not much I can do, really. I've just been lying here . . . th inking . . . thinking about my life . . . thinking about how close I came to . . . you know."

"Yes, I guess it was a bit of a shock. It certainly gave all of us a scare."

"Hmm, suddenly what I've been talking about with Brenda and Leo, our conversations about death, have become incredibly real and . . ."

" . . . you know my feelings about that . . ."

" . . . but these conversations have been important for me. When I look back on my life, I see how I've managed to avoid thinking about death; well, actually, I was just too focused on home and work life, and I simply pushed any concerns about death to the back of my mind. It's only over the past few months that I've taken the trouble to think about it. And now this happens . . . and, I must say, it's really muddled up what I was thinking previously."

Mandy stared out of the window and fidgeted as though she was debating whether to leave. "How's that?"

"I'm not sure where it's heading, but since coming in here, I have this sense that our talks have been a bit abstract, a bit cerebral. Now, suddenly, death, as it appears in my life, is solid and undeniably real. My brush with death came as a loud thud. An unmistakable signal . . . but one I can't put into words."

"We certainly didn't see it coming."

"I feel as though I've reached out and touched death, and, like a mari-nade, its sticky presence has spread and soaked through everything around me." He glanced up at Mandy's face and noticed her discomfort. "I'm sorry. You don't need to stay here listening to an old man's rambling thoughts."

"Stan, I'm always interested in what you have to say." She stood up and clasped his hands. "But, I'm afraid, I must go. I only arranged an hour off work."

Stan, now in his eighties, knew in his head that dying was approaching, and this had encouraged him to read and talk about it. His discussions with Leo regarding Heidegger had introduced him to the idea of finitude, but he had felt uncomfortable with confining it to a concept. He sensed it involved something more.

A number of thinkers besides Heidegger have adopted finitude in its varying guises to refer to the ways we, as individual beings, are held in place by a complex of intersecting constraints and limitations. Some thinkers have used finitude to emphasize more specific aspects of our boundedness. For example, Jean-Luc Nancy (2003) and Roger Frie (2013) have used it to refer to what limits and constrains consciousness.[3] Similarly, John Sill (1980) and David Weiss (2014) have focused on its function with developmental aspects that occur in the later stages of life.[4] Others, such as Françoise Dastur (1996) and Sami Pihlström (2016), have linked it more closely with the nature of human mortality[5]; others, such as Jan-Olav Henrikson (2011) and Arjan Markus (2004), have examined its function in religion[6]; others, such as Francesco Adorno (2010) and Alejandro Vallega (2009), have explored its role in artistic expression[7]; and still others, such as Irvin Yalom (2010) and myself (Adams 2018),[8] have explored the part finitude plays during critical moments in the course of one's life.[9]

Stan's life-threatening encounter had alerted him to the presence of fin-itude in every corner of his life. He sensed it as a suffusion that thoroughly permeated all aspects of experience. He encountered this at several levels si-multaneously: as an idea, as a sensation, and as an emotional connection, but no one level captured what it meant for him; rather, he experienced it as an intuition combining all three.

"Hi Stan," greeted Leo as he bounded into the ward. He helped Stan prop himself up with an extra pillow then sat in the chair by his bed. "Have they been treating you well?"

"As well as you'd hope."

They chatted for a while about the ward staff, about progress with Leo's study, and about events at home.

Eventually Stan switched to the topic he really wanted to discuss. "You remember the talk we had about Heidegger and his concept of finitude? Well, lying here following my close call with death, I've been thinking more about it . . . and I see it differently now. I now see finitude as permeating everywhere; its energy flows through all things."

"Yeah, you're saying the same thing as what I was saying before. Finitude constantly signals the intrinsic nature of my mortality."

"No, no, you're talking about it purely at a conceptual level. What's happened to me has convinced me it's more than that—much more. What's at stake is more than a dimension or condition for my existence. It's a dynamic process that, like swimming in a river, pushes and jostles me at every moment; it keeps flowing and flowing around me; a constant flow of energy that calls out and engages me as a whole."

"A constant, flowing energy?" queried Leo. "I don't understand."

"What I'm saying is that coming close to death has helped me appreciate—in my head, in my heart, and in my guts—the ever-present reality and nature of death. This isn't just an intellectual exercise. You can't even capture it with concepts."

"So you're pulling rank? You're claiming you're more qualified to talk about death than me?"

"Kind of . . . no," said Stan as he shuffled higher into his pillow. "All I'm saying is my close call with death has activated something inside of me; it's awoken something in me that has been hibernating for a very long time. But it involves far more than a shift in perspective."

Perhaps what Stan was talking about here approaches what the German philosopher Max Scheler had in mind when he talked about "an intuitive knowledge of mortality."[10] Scheler (1911) claimed that

Thus every first-hand life experience appears to us against the backdrop of a vital unit, temporally circumscribed before and after, which is present as such in every experience.[11]

Scheler was suggesting that mortality (and its connection to finitude) is embedded in the very nature of experience, which means that we, as experiencing subjects, can access it at any time in the form of an intuition. While as an intuition it is constantly available, perhaps because of the negative associations of finitude and death, we repeatedly put it to one side.

Finitude Marking

The English poet William Wordsworth penned an ode that he titled, *Intimations of Immortality from Recollections of Early Childhood*, in which he claimed, "To me the meanest flower that blows can give / Thoughts that do often lie too deep for tears."[12] His idea of immortality was associated with the wondrous way in which natural beauty affects the soul. He recognized how this volatile and amorphous engagement does not lend itself to being directly observed or talked about; rather, it is referenced indirectly in the form of hints and intimations. But this indirect referencing can be equally applied to personal mortality. My-death and its various links with finitude are difficult to both think and talk about.[13] There is no clear object or event as there is when other people die. Like immortality, mortality does not lend itself to direct observation or clear expression. Instead we glean its presence through indirect hints and intimations, and from there we intuit the constant presence of my-death.[14]

Following on from this, the next question that springs to mind is this: If my-death—and its associations with finitude—are only indirectly accessed, how are these intimations achieved? What are the mechanisms whereby they are inculcated into our lives? To answer these questions, we need to look a little closer at how we engage with finitude.

The following discussion will argue that we become aware of our finite condition through signals that mark out our boundedness. These signals or markers are objects or events that have acquired links with the various ways we are constrained. But these marked links involve more than vague associations; they also bear with them significant and direct relationships with the conditions or activities that maintain relevant underlying constraints. They have, one could say, an immediate connection that is clearly linked to real consequences for what determines our boundedness.

To illustrate this point further, consider the symbol of a ticking clock as it is used to represent elapsing time. Contrast this with the way celebrating a birthday marks the elapsing of another year of a person's life. To be sure, symbols of the passing of time are tangled up in the ceremony of birthdays, including such events as the burning of candles, joking about aging, and clapping to represent each passing year. The generalized signals of the passage of time, in this case the birthday cake, adds some emphasis to the marker. But the event itself, the anniversary, marks something real; namely, the reality of the elapsing of time. The immediacy of the link is important. While someone might appreciate the lighting of a cake and singing happy birthday six months after the date, it holds little potency in terms of marking the passing of time itself. When such objects are employed to directly mark an event of significance, the process attains a level of meaning and intensity that takes it well beyond mere symbolization. What is important is that marking the event connects in some specific and direct way to something else of key significance, in this case the person's date of birth.

Other events and contexts can function as common markers of finitude. It can be seen in the celebration of major milestones, such as an anniversary or a retirement; in acknowledging achievements, as occurs at prize-givings or graduations; and in the recognition of major transitions, such as naming a first child or signing divorce papers. Some of these events are particularly potent markers of finitude. For example, a funeral marks the end of a person's life and indirectly marks the prospect of death for those attending. More commonly, finitude is marked by small and often variable associations that can act cumulatively to highlight one aspect of personal limitation. For example, the finite nature of a person's lifespan is often marked by body changes over time: for women such changes might be marked by the end of fertility at menopause or the appearance of unwanted wrinkles; for men, key markers could be balding and graying hair, reduced flexibility and dexterity, and losses in strength and stamina. Such marking also occurs with physical and social contexts. Our position in space is often marked by objects such as road milestones, hill monuments, and church spires; our position in social contexts is often marked by symbols of allegiance—such as team uniforms, clothing fashions, wedding rings, and tattoos—and status signifiers—such as badges, medals, and expensive jewelry.[15]

In a similar fashion, the specific changes to our bodies as we get older go further than symbolizing our approaching old age; they serve to mark actual and important limitations and boundaries. For example, the way joints creak in an aging body does more than symbolize aging; it is a real event with real implications and real significance for the person concerned. Similarly, a man having a vasectomy might respond strongly to how it marks changes in his life. For him, his vasectomy might mark the end of a phase in his life. Perhaps it marks the passage from his years of reproductive potential into that uncertain world of impotency that is associated with old age. It might also signal deeper anxieties about becoming less sexually active or, perhaps more importantly, about becoming perceived as less of an object of sexual desire. The vasectomy, in an immediate and specific way, marks a transition point which has solid biological consequences that extends well beyond merely symbolizing aging.[16]

As these examples suggest, the two key aspects that enable signs, objects, and events to function as markers of finitude are the qualities of the markers—and all they signal—and the reality to which they are connecting. It is this pairing of sign with reality that activates an emotional, almost visceral sense of connection. The linkage is intuited more than thought; its potency lies more in the way it speaks to the heart.

Stan liked the way the morning sunlight danced on his bedroom wall. He was watching its changing form as the sun rose further and cast images lower down.

It was now two days since his return home, and a visiting nurse was busy dressing the wound from his operation. While he was disappointed that he had to stay in bed for two weeks, he was still very pleased to be home and surrounded by familiar objects.

Leo sauntered into the room and peered over the nurse's shoulder. "Ooh, that wound . . . still a bit nasty. But I can see it's closing up nicely. How's it feeling?"

"Ah, well," replied Stan, "I can put up with the pain and discomfort, but I don't like what it's telling me."

The nurse closed Stan's pajama shirt and drew up his blanket. "There, all good 'til tomorrow." She tidied up her equipment and walked out of the room guided by Winston.

"Okay, Stan, describe to me what the wound's telling you?"

"It's a wound now, but soon it will form into a permanent scar." With effort he pulled his blanket up to his neck. "And from now on, whenever I look at it, it will remind me of this major change in my life." He paused and glanced again at the sunlight on the wall. "See, the doctors told me my heart's permanently damaged; that it's running only on half its capacity. And that means there's lots of things I won't be able to do."

"But there will also be lots of things you can do?"

"Okay, but at the moment I'm focused on what I'm losing. I can't help it," stated Stan as he closed his eyes. "I won't be able to do things in the garden like I used to; things like digging holes, lifting heavy pots, and hoeing out weeds; all essential for keeping a garden operating. I won't be able to go hiking anymore, just short walks without any exertion. I'll probably need someone to help me with the shopping. I won't be. . . ."

"Okay, okay, I get it. That scar will be the emblem of these new limitations."

"Precisely; its permanence is yelling deeply into my soul, 'you are finite' and 'you only have one life to live.' It feels as though a noose is slowly tightening around me, squeezing my neck, restricting me . . . and there's no escape."

" 'Noose'? What, a noose around your neck?" queried Leo staring at him with an alarmed expression. "Don't tell me you're looking for an exit?"

"No, no . . ." said Stan. "On the contrary. What I'm getting at is how these events not only signal things are winding down, that I'm getting closer to dying, but they link up with all the other things that limit me . . . you know . . . all the other signals that tell me I'm finite."

Leo smiled, both relieved that Stan was not considering an exit and bemused at the role reversal with him asking rather than being asked about suicide. "So you're saying all these many signals of your finitude act as constant reminders of death. They allow death to beam into and shine onto everything that is happening to you."

"Yes, but it's more than an intellectual realization. Look, at the moment I'm lying here prone. I can't move or do anything. My life is severely constrained, so I'm totally immersed in what it means to be finite." Stan wiped away the small beads of sweat from his forehead. "I'm fully in touch with my finitude, but in this I realize I could be in touch with it at any time; reminders of finitude are always present; I've just failed to switch into seeing them and in appreciating what they are saying."

Leo expressed concern that Stan's talk of an "exit" signaled an interest in some form of suicide. Recent debates on the ethics of euthanasia and physician-assisted suicide have led to considerable discussion in the media, scholarly journals, and medicine. However, these debates have focused mainly on the question of autonomy about the timing of dying and these considerations have eclipsed issues associated with my-death.[17]

Stan, for his part, was not thinking of taking control of his final end; rather, he was focused on the ways finitude markers had intensified his appreciation of life. He described how the scar from his operation would, from then on, mark his close call with death, but he used it only as an exaggerated example of how we might manage to connect with finitude all the time. The markers are there; we just need to attend to them. Moreover, he was claiming that my-death is not accessed by thinking; rather, it is signaled by the way finitude is marked in our everyday lives, such that what is required is a shift in orientation, an opening up of mind, heart, and inner being to finitude and its constant signaling of the reality of my-death.

Brenda knocked on Stan's door and was greeted by the nurse leaving after she had dressed his wound. She strode through and sat in the armchair facing Stan's bed. She talked over Stan's progress with his recovery before resuming their favorite topic. "So, tell me, how has having the operation shifted your views on death?"

"Well, as I might have told you in hospital, I reckon throughout life death has been reaching out to me, trying to tell me it's there and constantly inviting me into its presence. What I've come to realize is its presence in finitude runs through so many things. Finitude has been sending out signals, continually transmitting death to me, in the form of both little signals and big signals, and I've just not been tuning in."

"Signals? Like what?"

"Well, um . . . in a kind of big way—and this goes on continuously— concerns memory. As I grow older my memories slip away. I remember less and less of the detail of what things were like when I was twenty. This, when you think about it, is a kind of death. I know there are many people and many events that I can no longer recall. Those memories have gone, and gone for good, and those many people and events from the past have dissolved into the ether; their memory has faded just like a photograph left in the sun."[18]

"I don't think forgetting only happens when you're older," commented Brenda thoughtfully. "I can't remember half the people in my class at high school, and I wouldn't recognize them if I passed them in the street. So, in a sense, they're dead to me. This keeps happening all through life."

"Yes, you're right. Time keeps erasing many things that were once important in our lives."

"Okay, Stan, now, what are some of the little ways death signals itself?"

"That's just what I was speaking to Leo about a couple of days ago: that finitude is marked all around through the various ways we are bounded and constrained. For instance, I'm constrained by my body; as it ages I'm less able to do things; I can't run and jump as I once did. I am reminded of this whenever I struggle on-board a bus or fail to open a jar. I sense the limitations in my creaking bones."

"I see; so each time you detect a limitation, it reminds you of your broader finite existence, and this connects you with death."

"Yes, sort of, but it's more than a matter of thinking; like I sense it more than think it. Indeed, I'm more aware of it in my guts than my head."

Brenda glanced across and could see that the bags under Stan's eyes were swelling. Despite his enthusiasm for the topic, he was tiring. "Stan, I think I should be off. I can see you're needing some rest."

Stan looked disappointed but nodded his agreement. "Brenda, before you go, can you go over to that set of drawers in the corner; yes, those ones. Open the top drawer and on the left hand side you'll see a set of keys on a brown keychain. Please take these back with you and anytime you or Mandy or Leo want to visit or to check up on me, please feel free to let yourself in."

"Thanks. That sounds sensible. It'll save you having to answer the door."

So death, in its form as my-death, asserts its presence through its contribution to finitude markers. In this way, a potent finitude marker could also act as an indirect marker of my-death. For example, a close call during a car accident or an operation, besides signaling the limitations of bodily existence, could also signal the close proximity of my-death. This is not a thought response; rather it occurs more as a thud from inside that drums out the inevitability of dying.

My-Death Everywhere

Stan had proposed that we live constantly surrounded by markers of finitude which, each in its own way, transmits reminders of our mortality. He also proposed that intuitions of finitude enable us to embrace my-death. The early twentieth-century Bohemian-Austrian poet and novelist Rainer Maria Rilke said as much when he claimed

Death is our friend precisely because it brings us into absolute and passionate presence with all that is here, that is natural, that is love . . . . Life always says Yes and No simultaneously. Death (I implore you to believe) is the true Yea-sayer. It stands before eternity and says only: Yes.[19]

According to the passionate suffusion frame, finitude markers signal how my-death saturates every moment and infuses everything around with its presence. It is signaled in many endings: the last drop from a bottle of wine, the last leaves to fall in autumn, the end of school, the end of a marriage. It is also signaled, strangely enough, by many of the beginnings: the first wrinkles, the first hair loss, and the decade birthdays—fifty, sixty, seventy, eighty. Both endings and beginnings signal my finite being as well as signaling the force of my-death standing behind them.

Brenda used the spare keys Stan had given her to let herself in and then to settle into the chair by his bed. "I've been thinking more about what you were saying, and I'd be interested in you talking more about how you see death everywhere."

Stan lifted himself slightly and turned onto his side. "Well, it's a bit of a work in progress."

"That's okay. It's dove-tailing with my work in progress."

"I've been thinking back over how it's functioned in my life. Before now, I had no idea about finitude, but, looking back, I think I had some intuitive sense of it. First, back to when I was an adolescent, a young hooligan driving fast around our neighborhood, I used to seek out opportunities for danger; you know, spinning out in cars, drinking excessively, picking fights, all manner of dangerous activities . . . we just seemed to constantly crave to be close to death. We used to play this game called 'chicken' where two cars drove as fast as they could toward each other daring the other to be the first to pull out. It's a wonder any of us survived."

"I don't remember anything like that."

"Maybe it's a guy-thing," commented Stan. "Then, in the military, when I did my first tour in Vietnam, there I didn't need to chase reminders of finitude anymore; every day was full of them; all us soldiers bathed in their constant presence: at any moment we could have been blown up or shot by a sniper; we could sense these possibilities all around; they constantly kept us connected to the vibrancy of death."

"Oh, come on, that must have been absolutely terrifying?"

"It was, but exhilarating at the same time. Then, when I returned to living a normal life in suburbia, working in a nine-to-five job, I didn't miss the fear and chaos of war, but I did miss all those regular signals of finitude that kept me in touch with death. In normal living, the signals were much weaker, and death seemed to fade away, leaving only a faint trace. This I found deeply troubling. I couldn't work it out; it seemed as though there was no friction in my life, and I needed to find something hard and tough to give my life traction. I felt constantly restless, always looking out for new opportunities, searching for more meaningful engagements, continually moving on."

"Did any of it come your way?"

"Sometimes. What I slowly realized was that it had less to do with what was happening outside me and more to do with what was going on inside." He laid his head back on the pillow and stared at the ceiling. "In hindsight, what I think was going on was a failure to recognize how much finitude runs through everything. I was waiting for it to come to me, rather than reaching out and trying to connect to it. So I made a point of looking out for and embracing all my boundaries and constraints. The more I did this, the more opportunities seemed to pop up. It wasn't just the obvious moments, like someone dying, but I found I could appreciate death in quiet moments such as walking along a beach or watching a sunset."

"Yes, I know what you mean. I sometimes get in touch with my mortality when I'm all by myself in very private moments. I remember sitting on a cliff one evening, and I had a sudden sense of the presence of death."

"Anyway, I settled down in this house and lived a routine and contented life . . . that was until it was all disrupted again in my late fifties. I guess what happened was I started to notice signs of my aging; you know, some balding, more wrinkles, less agility. . . . Death all of a sudden seemed to be rushing toward me, and I hadn't achieved half of what I wanted to out of life. It freaked me out, and I started doing very silly things, like buying a powerful motorbike and wearing inappropriately flashy clothes."[20]

"Hmm," responded Brenda thoughtfully. "For us woman our bodies provide us with more regular reminders of mortality; you know, with menstruation, child birth, and then menopause, then all the complications from these. I think we're more in touch with the physical reality of mortality than are men."

"Yes, maybe us men are more prone to pretending we're immortal because we have fewer biological reminders until we get old. And maybe that's why it hit me so hard all of a sudden."

"Here's another thing from a woman's perspective," said Brenda. "During my nursing training, I worked for a few months in a birthing ward. I remember watching in sheer wonder as each baby came into the world. It struck me then, as it does now, that being aware of my origins in birth, my genesis, is somehow similar to being aware of my mortality. They both seem connected to the same source."

"That's an interesting observation," said Stan. "Hmm, so it's not just the links of finitude to death, but it's also the way it links to our birth which also underpins its power. A very interesting idea, and yet another way in which finitude expresses itself."

Brenda's point echoes suggestions of what other authors have written about finitude. The German philosopher Hannah Arendt introduced the concept of "natality" as the human condition as "each newcomer possesses the capacity of beginning something anew."[21] Each birth is a wonder of creation that signals the source and power that lies behind its occurrence.[22] The French thinker Jean-Luc Nancy further underlined this idea by referring to it as "natal finitude."[23] The American philosopher Anne O'Byrne (2010) drew on both Arendt's and Nancy's ideas and developed her analysis of natality as contributing at a similar level as my-death to our sense of finitude.

> If the event of my birth is consigned to the past, there does indeed seem to be little reason to fear it, and certainly no reason to have any particular response to the eons of nonexistence that preceded it. After all, the well-known example is not wrong: we would all be more concerned if, waking in a hospital bed, we were told that we would have a moderately painful procedure the following day than if we heard that we had had an extremely painful one the day before. However, this also misses the point I am after. Death may be an event in my future, but I experience my mortality today. My birth may have happened years ago, but natality is a feature of my existence now.[24]

O'Byrne argued that mortality is but one side of what it means to be finite and that natality is another key element. Perhaps, as Brenda suggested, finitude can be viewed as sitting at one corner of a triangle with mortality and natality at the other corners.

To summarize, Stan's heart attack had triggered a reappraisal of his views about my-death which had helped him focus his previously meandering thoughts on the topic. He agreed with Leo that contact with my-death occurs indirectly through contact with finitude but, instead of viewing finitude as a necessary structural feature of existence, he viewed it more as a vital force in its own right. His brush with death had alerted him to the ways finitude was being signaled through a wide variety of what he identified as finitude markers. These markers included aspects of his position in time and place, his confinement in an aging body, and other limitations associated with personality, viewpoint, and culture. He saw these markers as so common that, if he maintained his awareness of them, then finitude, along with its relationship with my-death, could be maintained as a constant presence. This presence allowed him to build up a more intimate and personal relationship with my-death, instead of what he saw as the sterile structural relationship that Leo was proposing.

In addition to this, Stan's heart attack impacted on the others around him. Mandy, for instance, found his close call with death unnerving, particularly when she had invested so much energy in not talking about death. In a world surrounded by reminders of death, it took energy to maintain such silence, especially when surrounded by others who persisted in talking about it. Stan, her long-term friend and neighbor, nearly died. How could she continue to ignore what this means? Events were priming Mandy for a change.

Mandy called in on Stan to find him lying on the couch in the living room behind an assortment of books and magazines piled up on his coffee table. "I'm going to the supermarket and just wanted to check if there's anything you'd want. Any food or groceries?"

He smiled warmly on her entry. "No, my little team of visitors attend to all that." He propped himself up on a pillow. "But look, come and sit down in my comfy armchair and tell me about what's been happening for you lately."

"Oh, that's not very interesting. . . . Working in the shop, house work, you know." She settled into the armchair. "No, I'm more interested in your progress. You're looking much better."

"Yes, I'm doing well; my wound's healing, I'm awake more, and I'm feeling more energetic."

"I'm pleased to hear that Stan." She paused thoughtfully, then said tentatively, as though confessing a crime, "Actually, Stan, there is something I'd like your views on. Last night I had the weirdest dream. I don't usually remember dreams, but this one was so vivid it stayed with me well after I woke up." She paused again to study Stan's expression. "I dreamed I saw Maurice walking toward me down a long corridor. He was dressed in a white robe that kind of glowed as he walked. I waved at him but he just kept walking until he was only a few feet in front of me."

"Your Maurice? But he died over twenty years ago," he said, pausing to consider what this might mean. "So, at that point, did he say anything?"

"He looked directly into my eyes and—this is a bit strange—his mouth wasn't moving but I could hear his voice clearly in my head. He said, 'Don't worry, Mandy, Leo will be okay.' He repeated this a few times. Then he said, 'I have seen his future.' Then he turned and left." She shrugged. "What do you make of that?"

"Hmm, the dream seems to be telling you to stop worrying about Leo dying. What do you think?"

"Same. But there's two things here. The dream suggests that Maurice still exists in some form somewhere, and suggests that both Leo and I will exist similarly after we die. This is reassuring. But the dream also seems to be suggesting that death isn't really a big deal; that it's not the big ogre I've made it out to be."

"I'd agree. It seems to be giving you permission to engage with death without too much worry."

"Oh Stan," said Mandy with her eyes welling and tears beginning to dribble down her cheeks. "I've been very silly imposing on everyone my worries about death and forbidding anyone from talking about it."

"No, I don't see that as silly," replied Stan with a reassuring smile. "Dying for everyone is scary. But death, particularly my death, well that's another matter. Since my heart attack, I'm more and more convinced that death is everywhere and that it is in our interests to reach out and draw it in close."

Mandy leaned forward in the armchair and wiped her tears away. "I can see what you're saying, but I'm not sure how to do that."

Stan's close call with death had unsettled Mandy's resolutely pragmatic approach to life. She could feel a storm was approaching but was unsure from whence it came.

Notes

1. P. Adams, *Navigating Everyday Life: Exploring the Tension Between Finitude and Transcendence* (Lanham, MD: Lexington Books, 2018).

2. For example, see Jan-Olav Henriksen's discussion of finitude in *Finitude and Theological Anthropology* (Leuven: Peeters, 2011).

3. J.-L. Nancy, *A Finite Thinking* (Stanford, CA: Stanford University Press, 2003) and R. Frie, "On the nature and meaning of human finitude," *American Journal of Psychoanalysis* (73, 158–72, 2013).

4. J. Sill, "Disengagement reconsidered: Awareness of finitude," *Gerontologist* (20:4, 457–62, 1980) and D. Weiss, "What will remain when we are gone? Finitude and generation identity in the second half of life," *Psychology and Aging* (29:3, 554–62, 2014).

5. F. Dastur, *Death: An Essay in Finitude* (London: Athlone, 1996) and S. Pihlström, *Death and Finitude* (Lanham, MD: Lexington Books, 2016).

6. J. -O. Henriksen, *Finitude and Theological Anthropology*, and A. Markus, *Beyond Finitude* (Frankfurt: Peter Lang, 2004).

7. F. Adorno, "Against posthuman ideology: Aesthetics and finitude of the individual," *Res: Anthropology and Aesthetics* (57/58, 344–54, 2010), and A. Vallega, *Sense and Finitude* (Albany: State University of New York Press, 2009).

8. I. Yalom, *Staring at the Sun: Overcoming the Terror of Death* (San Francisco: Jossey-Bass, 2010), and P. Adams, *Navigating Everyday Life*.

9. In *Navigating Everyday Life*, I examine the role of finitude in both daily life and in moments of crisis and transition. I describe its action as involving a multidimensional grid of interlocking coordinates. These coordinates—situation, body, person, and outlook—combine through every moment at one intersection point to condition each moment of experience.

10. For more discussion on Scheler, see B. Schumacher, *Death and Mortality in Contemporary Philosophy* (Cambridge: Cambridge University Press, 2010).

11. Quoted in a footnote by B. Schumacher, *Death and Mortality*, p. 59, and translated from Scheler's *Tod und Fortleben* (1911–14) p. 23.

12. W. Wordsworth, *Ode: Intimations of Immortality from Recollections of Early Childhood* (Boston: D. Lothrop & Co., 1884) p. 40.

13. For example, the unthinkable nature of finitude in its relationship to personal mortality is discussed by F. Dastur in *Death: An Essay in Finitude*.

14. See D. Krell, *Intimations of Mortality* (University Park: Pennsylvania State University Press, 1986), where he discusses Heidegger and finitude and cleverly titled his book accordingly.

15. These examples describe events where objects presented together form associations. Of course, the processes of marking in language play an important role in the rhetorical dimensions of how we speak. Marking is also related to one of the most important rhetorical tropes: metonymy. See R. Dirven and R. Porings, eds., *Metaphor and Metonymy in Comparison and Contrast* (Berlin: Mouton de Gruyter, 2002).

16. The psychological and emotional complexities involved in vasectomies are explored further by R. Cragun and E. Sumerau "Losing manhood like a man" *Men and Masculinities* (20:1, 98–116, 2017).

17. This topic extends into many other areas in addition to my-death, as described in Robert Weir's edited collection, *Physician-Assisted Suicide* (Bloomington: Indiana University Press, 1997). For a broader discussion on this issue, see T. Szasz, *Fatal Freedom: The Ethics and Politics of Suicide* (Syracuse, NY: Syracuse University Press, 2002).

18. Discussion of the existential impacts of memory loss are discussed by S. Ceci and U. Bronfenbrenner, "On the demise of everyday memory: 'The rumors of my death are much exaggerated' (Mark Twain)," *American Psychologist* (46:1, 27–31, 1991).

19. R. M. Rilke, "Letter to Countess Margot Sizzo-Noris-Crouy, Epiphany," in J. Macy & A. Barrows (eds, trans). *A Year with Rilke* (New York: HarperCollins, 1923) p. 250.

20. I explore these types of finitude marking in "Oscillating imbalances: Responding to the existentials in major life transitions," *Journal of Social Work Practice* (31:3, 323–6, 2017).

21. Hannah Arendt, *The Human Condition* (Chicago: University of Chicago Press, 1958) p. 9.

22. Arendt's influences from Heidegger are discussed by R. Flores in "The capacity to begin: Arendt's concept of 'natality,'" *Threads* (3, 80–87, 2015).

23. Nancy outlined his thinking on finitude in *A Finite Thinking* and developed his concept of "natal finitude" in *Being Singular Plural* (Stanford, CA: Stanford University Press, 2000). Also see A. López and M. del Rosario in "'An infinite task at the heart of finitude," *CR: The New Centennial Review* (17:3, 21–42, 2017).

24. Anne O'Byrne, *Natality and Finitude* (Bloomington: Indiana University Press, 2010) p. 3.

8

Point-of-Transition

The third enabling frame repositions the event of my-dying from a final dramatic endpoint to a point at which a transition occurs from one kind of life to another, in particular a transition from existence as currently experienced into some form of afterlife. This point-of-transition perspective extends current individual existence out from its finite, constrained form into some kind of ongoing continuation, perhaps as a soul continuing to live on in heaven or as a reincarnated entity or as a transcendent self dispersed into the cosmos.[1] As explored in Chapter 4, expectations of living on after death can help in reducing anxieties about death and distract from worries about dying as a final end-point. Indeed, Leo repeatedly accused his mother of buying into notions of an afterlife as a way of avoiding or even denying the reality of my-death. He ridiculed her understanding as irrational and self-deluding.

Nonetheless, approaching continuation in an afterlife as an avoidance strategy misses out some of the wider and positive aspects offered by this frame. Belief systems that interpret death as a transition help to clear away many of the concerns we might harbor about uncertainty, loss, and pointlessness. For instance, it promotes a stronger sense of what might lie beyond my-death. Any lessening of these concerns then generates space for other relational opportunities: it can help us continue to pursue a meaningful relationship with loved ones who have passed away, it opens up the prospect of my future dead self maintaining a relationship with the world of those who are still living, and it reduces the clutter and confusion related to fearing death, thereby freeing us up for a more direct and focused relationship with my-death.

But before examining the broader advantages of a point-of-transition frame, something happened to Mandy that dramatically transformed how she understood the merits of this frame and the manner in which she engaged with my-death.

Mandy was making her way back from Stan's house following yet another protracted conversation about the meaning of his brush with death. It was late in the evening, the stars were twinkling clearly, and the moon had yet to rise.

She edged her way through the hole in the fence and walked across her backyard. It was a warm evening and the stars were twinkling confidently above so she sat down to admire them from the reclining chair in the yard.

She was aware of the silence all around, interrupted occasionally by the chirping of a nearby cricket. She was also aware of her head still churning from the many claims that Stan had been making about death. These thoughts slowly dissipated as she became captivated by the beauty of the night sky.

She let other thoughts come and go until she reached a point where she felt detached from what she was thinking. Her whole awareness was now focused on the piercing points of starlight held majestically against the deep blackness of the sky. Suddenly, without warning, she felt her consciousness being thrown into this blackness; it felt as though her whole being was becoming absorbed by all she observed, as though she had become one with the universe in its entirety.

She had never had an experience as intense as this before. She was feeling a range of intense emotions: joy, excitement, rapture. But the emotions weren't the most important part. What mattered was what this absorption, this intense sense of unity, was telling her. It was conveying to her that her life extended well beyond its current constrained and mortal form. Her particular existence and her death were only minor interruptions in this ongoing continuity. The truth of this was self-evident in itself, beyond any form of doubt and in no need of any further verification.

She wasn't sure how long this experience lasted; maybe five minutes, maybe half an hour. It left as quickly as it came. But that, too, didn't matter. What remained was the correctness of the experience; she was left with a confident sense that she had connected with the indescribable reality of a continuing presence; a presence that extended well beyond her current life.

She also recognized that it would be foolhardy to share this realization with other people. She needed time to process what it meant. She had no way of expressing to others the truth of what she had encountered, and there was a high chance that people would think she was crazy.

Mandy's mystical encounter with the night sky presented her with a way to feel more confident about life continuing after death.[2] It allayed many of her doubts, freed her from the terror of my-death, and allowed her to reappraise her relationship to it.

Life After Death

At this point it is important to understand why Mandy had clung so insistently to the idea of an afterlife and why she had consistently discouraged conversations about death.

Mandy carried the casserole pot over to the table and called out for Brenda to join her at dinner. Leo was out with friends, so it would give the two of them a chance to catch up.

Mandy opened the discussion. "You know how I've been asking you not to engage Leo in conversations about death. . . ."

"Oh, I'm sorry," interrupted Brenda. "I've tried to keep him off the topic, but . . . but he's very persistent. No really, I've tried to honor your request. Believe me. I have. . . ."

"No, no, Brenda, don't worry. I'm not going to tell you off." Mandy stretched her hand across the table and gently grasped Brenda's hand. "Truly, I'm not concerned with that anymore." She pulled her hand back but maintained a direct gaze into Brenda's eyes. "On the contrary, I want to apologize to you for giving you a hard time."

"Ah, I . . . " Brenda looked confused. "I don't understand. What made you change?"

"Well, I began shifting when talking to Stan. Our conversations and what has happened to him have led me to think quite differently about death. I now realize I got everything out of proportion and that death is a necessary part of life. For me it represents a very important transition point; a subject I would like to explore further." She sat back to study the surprised look on Brenda's face. "But I also want you to understand why it worried me."

Brenda leaned back in her chair, unconsciously mirroring Mandy's posture. "Okay, fire away."

"Well, it all began when Leo was about fourteen, when he started listening to heavy metal music. I thought it was just a passing fad, but then he started spending more and more of his time and money on this music. Have you heard it? It's pretty gross."

"I've seen these guys grunting into microphones with electric guitars blasting constantly. Never appealed to me."

"Me neither. But for him it was everything. He spent increasing amounts of time on the internet tracking down recordings and reading everything he could. He seemed totally obsessed, so I decided to look more closely at the material he was accessing. I found, to my horror, nearly all of it's about death. What's more, most of the imagery relates to death: skulls, skeletons, coffins, and graves. Added to this are all the instruments of death: scythes, swords, daggers, and even fancy guns." She leaned forward to eat more of her dinner. "You should have seen the posters he hung all over his walls; lurid images of screaming skulls and half-clad dying maidens. I dunno."

"Hmm, but don't you think all that's just part of an adolescent male's emerging sexuality? It's not going to last once he's immersed in a real sexual relationship."

"That's what I thought, or hoped," said Mandy. "But then I looked even closer at the images and reading materials and realized that much of it was subtly and often blatantly referring to suicide. More than that, it was casting suicide as a legitimate, even a noble exit."[3]

"Goodness, that's scary, your son being persuaded of the merits of killing himself."

"Yes, exactly; it scared the bejesus out of me," said Mandy raising her arms then leaning forward and looking straight at Brenda. "See, Leo is the main person in my life. If I lost him, I . . . I . . . well, I just wouldn't cope." She looked down to the table. "I didn't want to think about his death, or my death, or anyone's death. I just wanted the whole topic to go away. He's everything to me. I shudder each time he mentions death, and no matter what I try, I can't shake his interest in this topic."

The discovery Mandy made during her mystical experience invigorated her confidence in believing in some form of continuation after death. With my-dying seen as a point of transition, my-death carries less of a sting, and, accordingly, she found herself more relaxed about thinking and talking about it. Indeed, the conversation she was having with Brenda would not have been possible before this encounter.

"So what happened next?" asked Brenda, as she spooned more of the casserole onto her plate.

"Well, as you suggested, Leo's interest in heavy metal waned. No doubt he still listens to it but nothing like he did five years ago. Then, more recently, I kept hearing Leo saying that nothing exists beyond death; that annihilation was all we can look forward to. All my fears were reactivated."

"Yes, I can understand that."

"What's more," continued Mandy hesitantly, "I don't know if you've heard, but when Leo was only two, his dad, Maurice, who was working for the electricity company as a linesman, was severely electrocuted. Someone made a mistake with the circuit breakers, and he was the mug up the pole." She looked away, her face muscles straining against the pressure of tears. "He was taken to hospital, but his burns were too severe, and he died the next day."

"Oh, Mandy, I'm so sorry to hear that. It must have been devastating."

"Hmm, it was." Her chin quivered as she held back her tears. "It was like my whole world had fallen apart. Everything we had worked for was now in disarray. The worse thing was losing our future together; he and I would not be growing old together and watching our children grow up or, perhaps, watching them having children; we wouldn't be there together."

"I guess it would take some time to recover from such an unexpected loss?"

"But I had to be strong. I had to take care of my little boy. I had to find ways of bringing in money and keeping the home afloat." She put her knife and fork together and wiped her lips with a napkin. "And then, a year later, there was the inquest. More chaos and disruption. I felt constantly pulled apart."

"It must have been hard to stay strong with all that going on."

"To stay strong, I cut off emotionally from everything and everybody, including my friends. All I could cope with was the idea that Maurice was up in heaven looking down on me, encouraging me and approving of what I was doing, and that one day we would be reunited. This allowed me to carry on. We were only temporarily separated."

"I can see why you didn't like us talking about death."

"Yes, it was like pulling off a scab before the wound had healed." Mandy relaxed back into her chair. "See, whenever anyone talked about a person's death, or even anything to do with death, it all linked up with Maurice's death and that horrible time. Then, on top of that Leo kept on insisting death was the final endpoint. What he said filled me with dread; it suggested to me was I would never see Maurice ever again. I could not bear to think that way."

If the person who dies continues in some form, whether that be an ethereal disembodied presence or perhaps even embodied in another form, if that person persists, then the relationship with that person also persists. The continuation of the relationship was what was important to Mandy, even if it meant delaying direct contact until she died. The idea of eventually reuniting with her husband enabled her to carry on life without sinking into overwhelming grief.

The Austrian psychiatrist Sigmund Freud proposed that a belief in immortality was hardwired into our psyche:

> We cannot, indeed, imagine our own death; whenever we try to do so we find that we survive ourselves as spectators. The school of psychoanalysis could thus assert that at bottom no one believes in his own death, which amounts to saying: in the unconscious every one of us is convinced of his immortality.[4]

The impacts of believing in an afterlife on our lives have been explored in a variety of ways. Ethan Benore and Crystal Park (2004) summarized research into the beneficial effects of afterlife beliefs for those who have lost loved ones and claimed that research was suggesting that such beliefs help people cope better with their distress. In particular, it enables people to "confront death's inevitability more hopefully, thus decreasing the initial stress engendered by the death of a loved one."[5] Others have highlighted how believing in an afterlife can result in better general mental health. For example, in a national survey in the United States, Kevin Flannelly and colleagues (2006) found such beliefs were associated with less troubles across all six domains of mental health they measured.[6] In another US survey of terminally ill cancer patients, Colleen McClain-Jacobson and colleagues (2004) found such beliefs were associated with lower levels of end-of-life despair.[7]

However, the positive effects of believing in an afterlife have been challenged, particularly for older people. For example, Deborah Carr and colleagues (2014) focused on 210 bereaved people from a large study of older people in Detroit. They found afterlife beliefs "powerfully affect intrusive thoughts, or unwanted and uncontrollable thoughts about . . . death."[8] This can lead to distress, particularly for those who have shaky or unsure beliefs about an afterlife. They concluded that while such beliefs may have short-term benefits, over the longer term they might discourage the bereaved from exploring new relationships and activities.

Brenda cleared up the dishes while Mandy prepared two herbal teas, then they both retired to the comfort of the living room.

"But you said earlier," noted Brenda, "that all our talk of death has helped you change your position on there being an afterlife."

"No, I still believe in an afterlife, despite what Leo says," clarified Mandy. "But I have a whole new take on it." She carefully sipped the edge of the cup. "Stan helped me appreciate how I've been a bit ridiculous censoring talk about death; death is important, and I need to find some way of relating to it."

"You know, I agree with him. Death is part of life, and we should embrace it."

"And so, lately, I've made a point of opening up to it," she paused. "Then suddenly, a few nights ago, it came to me. If when people die you don't treat it as an endpoint, rather as a transition point, much of the weight of grief and despair we feel about death is lifted. And, as Stan says, death, particularly my death, is different than dying." She leaned forward in the armchair. "See, I just feel that . . . no, I know for certain that there is an afterlife and that when Maurice died, and when I die, and when Leo dies, something about all of us persists; some aspect of us carries on after death, maybe as an individual, maybe as a collective, and this makes it possible for us to continue having meaningful relationships with those who have passed on. I now accept this wholeheartedly; I can see it no other way. And with that in mind, I no longer see much point in worrying myself sick about death."

"So, you're saying, rather than denying or hiding from death, your belief in an afterlife has helped you engage with death?"

"Yes, precisely!" said Mandy. "By fully embracing the idea of continuing after death, my worries and concerns about death are cleared away . . . well, at least put on hold. . . . If I know we will be carrying on in some form and that our relationships persist, then dying becomes less of an issue. And this frees me up to build up my relationships both with those who have gone before and with my own death. It allows me to focus in a much clearer way just on the nature of what my death means and to talk to people about it as we are doing now."

"Hmm, but surely it doesn't reduce your fears about the way you might die? You know, fears of pain and disablement . . . having to say goodbye?"

"No, but I think it will make that sort of distress more purposeful. It also helps me put my areas of worry into separate boxes: in this box I worry about loved ones dying, in this box I worry about me dying, in this box

I worry about death in general, in this box. . . . Well I'm just able to separate them out, and this means I can think about my own death in a less cluttered and less terrifying way."

Here Mandy explained how her strengthened belief in life after death had resulted in a number of changes that included a reduced fear of death, a lessening of the pain of losing a loved one, and a willingness to think and talk about my-death. K. Mitch Hodge (2011), a philosopher of mind from the United States, has explored other common ways these beliefs integrate into the lives of those who hold them. He focused particularly on the social benefits, stating that

> those who populate the afterlife are those individuals that matter to ourselves and our society. We imagine their continued existence in the afterlife in a way which permits a continued social exchange. . . . Since we understand death as an absence, we think about our deceased loved ones in [the] same way we would about a living but absent individual. . . . We continue to think about deceased individuals and, in turn, they continue to affect our thoughts, emotions and behaviors.[9]

Hodge viewed this as generating an imagined social world in which the usual social processes, such as mutual obligations and care, can continue and be further developed.

Research psychologists have turned their attention to the mental processes involved with afterlife beliefs. For example, Jesse Bering (2002) focused on how those who believed in an afterlife imagined the minds of dead people continuing to operate. He asked eighty-four US college students to read two types of stories at the end of which the main protagonist unexpectedly dies. Following this they were asked a series of questions regarding what they imagined was happening in the minds of the dead characters. He found surprising consistency in the way students responded. They more readily attributed dead characters with common everyday mental states (such as emotional or desire states) than those encountered less frequently (such as perceptual or psychobiological states). Bering argued this makes sense because

> we know what it is like, for example, to have our vision occluded and subsequently not to be able to see anything, we are able to call upon those experiences of absence and more effectively represent the mental ability to see

as ending at death than, say, the ability to think, which no sentient person has ever consciously been without.[10]

Other psychological studies have explored how people might antici-pate continuation after their own death. For example, Vera Pereira and colleagues (2012) interviewed forty young adult Portuguese afterlife believers and nonbelievers regarding how they would imagine their own dead selves (their "dead-I"). They, too, found reasonable consistency, with both believers and nonbelievers tending to imagine "the state in which being dead as a condition in which the I continues to be experienced."[11] From this they argued that belief in an afterlife could be considered an "in-tuitive religious concept" perhaps inbuilt into how we experience life.

Staying Connected

In the point-of-transition frame, the central idea of the afterlife can take on a variety of forms and functions. For some believers, the afterlife is seen as a real space inhabited by lovedones who are capable of communicating with us in various ways. For others, transitions into the afterlife can be followed by other transitions such as further reincarnations or arriving at different levels in heaven. For Mandy the true nature of the afterlife was still a mystery. All she was sure about was its existence as a place where loved ones went after death and where she would ultimately arrive.

Mandy unlocked Stan's kitchen door and was surprised to find him sitting upright at the table eating breakfast. "Stan, you're up!"

"Yes, I'm moving around a bit now. . . . But, sadly, my little helper makes sure breakfast isn't like it was before: no bacon, no butter; just muesli, fruit, and yoghurt."

"Never mind. I must say you're looking a lot healthier for it," said Mandy as she sat down opposite him.

"Yep, well, having nearly died, everyone's now going to great lengths to make sure I don't do it again." His initial smile gave way to a look of con-cern. "I'm sorry, I'm on that topic again. I don't want to talk about this if it upsets you."

"No, I'm okay. I really do want to speak about it now. Actually, thanks Stan; our conversations have helped lead me to finding a way of doing that."

"Hmm, that's good." He finished his last spoonful of muesli. "You know, I had a period in my late forties when thoughts of death troubled me. Looking back I guess it was some sort of mid-life crisis. I became deeply concerned about whether there was more to life than working and existing; whether there was any meaning beyond my mundane repetitive routines."

"I think we've all have times like that."

"Yes, but this was really intense. I couldn't stop fretting about it, and it kept me awake at night. I was searching for something, but I didn't know what. I felt there must be some greater purpose. So I started reading books about religion. Initially I read some Christian writers, like Richard Bucke and Thomas Merton.[12] But, interestingly, they led me to the great eastern religions, particularly Hinduism and Buddhism. There I discovered a whole new complex world of beliefs with many different schools and factions." Winston trotted over to Stan for a pat before curling up next to the table. "Like in Eastern religions, life is seen as eternally recurring. Death isn't important in itself. It has no finality."

"I'd be interested in their ways of thinking about the afterlife."

"Goodness, there's so many versions."[13] He scratched his head. "Tell you what, I'll talk a bit about Hindu beliefs, just as an example."

Mandy nodded her head expectantly.

"From what I remember," he continued, "Hindus see the mortal world as ruled by death, or Kala, who is a manifestation of Brahman himself. Brahman is the big guy, he represents the universal principle or ultimate reality of all existence. So death in its connection with Brahman is seen as part of the order of things; it is a transition point in the ever-cycling process of birth and death which makes up Samsāra and which forms the basis for one's Atman, or true self, which is destined to be reincarnated."

"I'm not familiar with all of these terms. It sounds complex. I learned about souls going to heaven at our church's Sunday school, and I can see how this might connect a little with some of these ideas."

"Yes, I guess the main thing is that, when you die, that's not the end of you. Something else goes on after death."

The idea of the afterlife provides the base for cultural and religious narratives about the fate of the individual self after death.[14] Whether the protagonist in these narratives is a Christian "soul" or a Muslim "soul" or a Hindu "Atman" or a Māori "wairua," what is anticipated is a journey through death into another realm of being in which some connected form of identity persists. For some traditions, particularly those referring to a "soul," the identity of an individual self continues but in a modified form. For others, individual identity becomes absorbed into a collective identity in some form of universal mind or cosmic consciousness.[15]

Mandy returned home from Stan's house to find Leo at the kitchen table munching toast.

"Been to see Stan?" he inquired.

"Yes, he's much better now. He's walking around and doing things." She sat down opposite her son and studied his expression. "I spoke to him about what will happen to us after we die."

Leo stopped eating and stared intensely back at her. "What? You've spoken to him about death?"

"Yes, and about what happens afterward." She smiled at the stunned expression that had spread across Leo's face. "I just want you to know. I've shifted my approach to this stuff. Now I really want to talk about it."

"I can't believe you're saying this. . . . You're totally relaxed?"

"Not entirely relaxed, but comfortable enough to speak with you."

"You're not going to go nuts?" He shook his head in disbelief. "After all this time. . . . So what's changed?"

"Events have helped me reconsider how I look at death," she said while continuing to smile. "I've been thinking it all through, and I now truly believe there is a life after death and that you, your father, and I will be reunited after we have died."

"I wish I could share your confidence, but, I'm sorry, I reckon that's highly unlikely, if not impossible."

"Oh, come on," exclaimed Mandy. "You're taking such a negative position; you're not going to gain anything thinking that way."

"You know I don't believe in all that nonsense. There's just no solid scientific evidence that any form of life continues after death. If there is, we'd have heard about it by now."

"I wouldn't be so sure," said Mandy wondering what evidence she might produce. "Well, what about people who've had near-death experiences? You know, intense experiences following close calls with death that involve visions and spiritual encounters? They're really common, particularly for people in intensive care or having surgery."

"Hmm, yes, I've heard of them."

"From what I've read they include a wide range of experiences, some that involve looking down on yourself from outside your body, others that involve spiritual awakenings. But, in their most common form, people report feeling as though they're going down a dark tunnel toward a bright light. It feels vivid and real. And sometimes in this bright light they might see some sort of shiny figure, a being of light; perhaps they see it as God or Jesus."

"Sounds much like a hallucination to me."

"No, but these are different. The people are perfectly normal, and what's more they're a hundred percent confident that they've looked forward into the afterlife, and, following the experience, many go on to make big changes in their lives. Another thing, some have reported being in a near-death experience and not wanting to return to normal life and eventually only do so because they don't want to hurt their loved ones."

"But lots of other things could explain such experiences. Being close to death is very stressful, so surely people's brains are being affected. Moreover, such experiences can be caused by brain events like epilepsy or toxic drug reactions.[16] Also, I've heard the religious figures you think you're seeing in these visions vary according to your background; a Muslim sees Mohammad, a Hindu sees one of their gods. You can't be sure they're looking into an afterlife, just projecting out their own beliefs."

"But you can't be sure they're not."

In 1975, the American medical physician Raymond Moody coined the term "near-death experiences" to refer to what many of his patients were reporting following life-threatening incidents while hospitalized. After hearing accounts by more than a thousand patients he became convinced, by their sheer volume, that something was going on and that perhaps what patients were experiencing was providing them with some sort of glimpse into what life might be like after death. Following on from him, Kenneth Ring (1980), a psychologist and founding figure in research into near-death experiences, documented a wide range of different types of such experiences,[17] and his work stimulated ongoing investigation into many aspects of what might be going on.[18] For example, it prompted Bruce Greyson (1983) to develop a sixteen-item Near-Death Experiences Scale,[19] which was subsequently used for closer study of the types of people for whom and types of contexts in which such experiences are likely to occur. Through all this, one question stood out: In reality, how common are these experiences? This proved difficult to answer mainly because of variability in how they are understood in different locations and different cultures. Indeed, population surveys that asked people directly about whether they had ever had such experiences yielded rates varying from 4 percent in Germany to 8.9 percent in Australia to 15 percent in the United States.[20] However, all agreed that rates increased markedly for people who have had close brushes with death, whether that be during surgery or from a heart attack or from a serious accident. For this group, some estimates are as high as a third.[21]

Early research on the nature of near-death experiences led to what Michael Kinsella (2017) refers to as the "afterlife movement."[22] Starting in 1981, in the US state of Connecticut, the International Association for Near-Death Studies (IANDS) was formed, followed later by establishing its own academic journal (*Journal of Near-Death Experiences*) then a highly developed website, a video channel, and several social media platforms. While IANDS formally expresses neutrality on the question of whether near-death experiences provide contact with the afterlife, undoubtedly many of its members see these experiences as informative. For example, Pranab Bhattacharya (2013) has argued that the common nature and high intensity of these experiences, coupled with the extent to which they have been researched, points to "genuine evidence for a non-physical reality."[23] Others are more skeptical about whether they provide glimpses into the afterlife. Keith Augustine (2015) referred to them as "internally generated fantasies" with medical, psychological, and cultural influences contributing in various ways.[24]

"Okay, okay," continued Leo. "But no-one has really survived death—no-one's actually fully died then come back properly to life. Some people have come very close; like when someone is clinically dead, then gets revived, but they didn't fully die. That's because in reality it's an impossibility, a contradiction in terms; my death is a condition for me being alive."

"Look, I'm not saying that they live on in the same manner as we live now," stated Mandy, more than a little flustered by her son's persistence. "It's a different kind of living; a carrying on of a person's soul or spirit, or whatever concept you prefer."

"It seems to me," said Leo slowly and in a measured tone, "that it makes little sense to talk of a person continuing to live after death. You think about it. Surely the body doesn't persist. The body is still there when someone dies, and we can watch it gradually decay into a skeleton. So what exactly does carry on? Your mind? Let's just reflect on what that involves. Whichever way you look at it, our minds are tangled up with what's going on in our brains and with what's happening in our senses. When we die, both our brains and our senses cease to function; they no longer operate. So what sense does it make to have a bodiless mind? It would be floating around in a sea of nothingness?"

"But don't you have a sense that it carries on?" pleaded Mandy.

"No, I don't."

Mandy frowned. "Look, despite all your appeals to science and logic, you're actually in a minority. Most people I know have some sense of their lives continuing after death. What's more, as far as I can tell, science has given us very little insight into what it means to die."

"So it's best not to jump to conclusions."

"What I'm trying to get across to you is that there's really no evidence for what you're saying, that death is the end of everything. You're in the same boat as me, except, my approach is more hopeful and it allows me to believe in connection to people who have gone before."

Leo realized that, from his mother's expression, he may have pushed his point too hard. "Ah, Mom, I can see we're never going to see eye-to-eye." He paused. "But thanks for talking it over. You know, this is the first time we've been able to talk about this without getting upset."

Mandy chose not to contest the rationality of her position. She knew this would not get anywhere with Leo. Besides, she was now confident in her position, and convincing him was not so important. What she was seeking was some concession from him regarding the possibility of an alternative position.

Leo's arguments regarding the implausibility of life after death has been a topic of fierce philosophical debate. The history of Christian thinking has a long and rich heritage of discussion on the nature of the afterlife.[25] For example, Robert Almeder (1992)[26] argued that there is as much empirical evidence for personal survival after death as there is for the past existence of dinosaurs. Terence Nichols (2010) claimed that, even in the face of modern scientific thinking,

> we can still make a credible case for life after death with God, for a soul that survives bodily death, for bodily resurrection, and for heaven and hell.[27]

Nichols based his arguments on appeals to Christian theology. However, the language of heaven, souls, and eternity have proved less persuasive with many modern thinkers. For example, Benjamin Matheson (2017) argued that practical identity cannot continue after death because an integrated body and mind are conditions that enable individual identity to occur.[28] Michael Martin and Keith Augustine (2015) compiled a large collection of essays contending that life after death is a myth that lacks any reasonable empirical evidence or any coherent argument.[29] Andrew Eschleman (2016) approached this differently by arguing that the language used to discuss the afterlife has rhetorical or figurative elements that can have meaning and value while not really needing to believe literally in our lives continuing after death.[30]

In the end, Mandy concluded this debate was unresolvable. Neither Leo nor she was able to produce conclusive arguments either for or against. She preferred to believe in life after death because it provided her with a more positive outlook on her future, and she felt her position was shared with the majority of other people she knew. Indeed, her point has support in research. For example, Jean Twenge and colleagues (2016), in their General Social Survey of around 59,000 Americans, were able to compare responses to questions about spirituality over a forty-year period stretching back to 1972.[31] They found progressive drops in the number of people participating in spiritual practices such as attending religious services, believing in God, and praying. For example, those reporting they did not believe in God increased from 13 percent in 1989 to 22 percent in 2014. Contrast this with the opposite trend for people reporting belief in an afterlife, rising from 76 percent in 1974 to 79 percent in 2014. Two other aspects of these results are worth noting: those who reported never attending religious services but still believing in an afterlife more than doubled from 7 percent in 1974 to 15 percent in 2014, and younger people (18- to 29-year-olds) were more likely to report believing in an afterlife, 73 percent 1974 and 80 percent in 2014. So, despite overall drops in the number of people engaging in spiritual beliefs and practices, belief in an afterlife has proved remarkably resilient and, given the rises with younger and nonreligious people, looks likely to continue as such well into the future.

After-Death in Everyday Life

Mandy's reassertion of her core belief in life after death has strengthened her willingness to engage in an ongoing relationship with my-death, but how does her point-of-transition frame compare with the previous two frames, essential structures and intuitive suffusion?

Mandy brought Stan over some of her baked muffins and found him fixing a faulty lamp in the living room. She placed the plate of muffins on the sideboard then lowered herself on to his couch. "I've been talking to Leo about what happens after we die, and he's been bashing me over the head with science and philosophy. There's no way he's going to accept the idea of life after death."

Stan placed his tools back in his toolbox, looked up at Mandy, and nodded a grateful smile. "Thanks for the muffins." He walked across and settled into the armchair opposite her. "You're right, there's no way he'll see his death other than the end of everything."

"I wish he was open to other possibilities," she sighed. "It's such a morose way to look ahead. . . . But there's one point he did make that's got me thinking. He said an afterlife, whether that be an ongoing presence or a recurring cycle or whatever, that such a life could end up meaningless because it has no clear boundaries."

"Hmm, I'd say that is a bit of an issue, and one that occurred to me as well. See, if you take dying out of the equation—with you carrying on into an afterlife—then you lose the bite that gives your life form and meaning."

"But the 'bite,' as you call it, is still there. Daily life remains just as bounded and constrained as ever."

"No, but without my death lurking at the end of each boundary, boundedness loses its potency; finitude just hangs there stripped of its power; a boundary without the prospect of death is a far weaker boundary. I'd say that's why Leo is so adamant about death as a final ending. He sees it as an integral and necessary part of what it means to exist. You take death away, and it all falls apart."

"No, it doesn't, because death still hangs there; it's there as a point of transition. Admittedly, it's not as ominous as viewing death as nothingness, but it's still potently connected, but in a more positive way."

"Okay, what about the role of all those things and events that mark finitude? You know, the things like signs of aging and personal boundaries, which we've been calling 'finitude markers'? They only have potency because they're connected to something really powerful."

"Ah, but death as a point-of-transition is really powerful. For example, I don't have access to it, yet I know it lies ahead of me and will absolutely

change everything. I have no direct contact with anyone in the afterlife other than knowing it's there. That's really powerful in my book." She
picked some of the topping off her muffin. "My mother was Catholic, so
when I was a child I went to Catholic schools and every Ash Wednesday
the priest would put a cross made up of ash on our foreheads saying something like, 'remember that dust thou art, and to dust thou shalt return.' We
were literally marked by the inevitability of our death, and we carried that
mark around all day." Mandy paused and stared deeply into Stan's watery
eyes. "Dear Stan, you're always so kind and interested." She reached across
to gently clasp his wrinkled hands. "Up until recently I've been so afraid of
death and finitude for that matter. Now I feel more ready to engage with
finitude and its connections with my death. The afterlife doesn't wipe finitude out. These finitude markers are for me linked to the inevitability of
our transition from a bounded life into the afterlife. And I am now trying to
engage with these markers every day."

Mandy was responding to Stan's challenge that believing in an afterlife would result in finitude losing its force because my-death, as a final
end, would no longer be present. She pointed out that my-dying as a
point of transition is still a profoundly significant event, capable of char-
ging anything connected to it with potent meanings. Moreover, this potency is carried through to the various finitude markers which pepper
everyday life.

The way Mandy achieved this new engagement involved an interesting series of changes in her outlook. Prior to her mystical experience, her weaker
and more uncertain belief in an afterlife had generated ambivalence: on
the one hand, she subscribed to a belief in life after death, but, on the other,
she was never really sure. Even as a way of reducing her fear of death it was
only partially effective because worry from the uncertainty of her belief
counteracted any relief she gained from believing in continuation. It also
meant she was unresponsive to markers of finitude because they, too, had
formed associations with this ambivalence. After her mystical experience,
her deep engagement with my-dying as a point of transition had enabled
her, with absolute confidence, to connect with my-death. The afterlife was
there as a fact, which enabled the event of my-dying to take on a definite
form; a form certain and solid enough for her to hang things off. Finitude
markers also took on a definite form; she could relate to what constrained
and bounded her life because they were now linked to my-death as a point of

transition. Furthermore, since finitude markers were constantly surrounding her, she always had constant access to these linkages whenever she wanted, and, through these linkages, my-death was then able to mutate into the form of a constant companion.

On Mandy's return from next door she found Brenda reading at her usual place at the kitchen table. "Ah, Brenda, I've been chatting with Stan. He's coming up with some very stimulating ideas."

"Ah, yeah, I really like talking things over with him. Not bad for someone in his eighties."

Mandy sat down at the table opposite Brenda. "I've worked out why I find it so much easier than before to think and talk about death."

"You've certainly changed. Was it because of what Stan went through?"

"Well, only partially. It was more to do with a switch in me. Alongside my conviction that life continues after death came a willingness to embrace both my finiteness and my mortality."

"So you moved from a scared cat to a fearless lion."

"Hah, well, a little bit like that," laughed Mandy. "What I then found I could do was link the afterlife into daily life. See, my death is like the entrance way, the portal into the afterlife, so the two are very interconnected. And, as Leo reminds us, my death is also linked to everything that holds me as constrained and bounded in every moment throughout my life; in other words, it connects in a fundamental way to my finitude. Moreover, I'm constantly in touch with finitude; since finitude is marked in so many ways in my daily life, it's always there for me to access whenever I choose. So, across this chain of connections—markers-finitude-death-afterlife, and back the other way—the afterlife has become a constant presence in what I'm experiencing."

"Ah, so your sense of an afterlife becomes like a parallel dimension to what's going on around you," suggested Brenda.

"Yes, that's it, a parallel dimension; always there, and I can tune in and out of it as I choose." Mandy sat back in her seat and studied Brenda. "Don't any of your hospice patients talk of having a connection to the afterlife? I mean, it must be something that concerns them?"

"They certainly talk about what it might be like after they die, but they do it in lots of different ways. Some talk of fearing it, some look forward to it, some. . . ."

"What about you? Do you have a sense of a life after death?"

"I didn't used to, but now I don't know anymore. All this talk about death has muddled me up, and I'm afraid I don't know where I stand. The way you describe the afterlife does make me think I could approach it that way. But Leo's and Stan's approaches are also attractive." Brenda paused and stared down at her knuckles on the table. "But I just don't know anymore."

Earlier in the book, particularly in Chapter 4, belief in an afterlife was seen as a way to avoid thinking about my-death. This chapter has explored how a strong commitment to the central idea of the afterlife has the capacity to enable an ongoing relationship with my-death. Mandy's move from a soft to a firm belief in the afterlife effectively reduced her fear of death to a point where she could engage positively with the markers of finitude that signaled her death. By means of these constantly repeating linkages, my-death and the afterlife have become, in her words, like a dimension running alongside what she was experiencing. Brenda was the most recent person to discuss this with her, and now Brenda was wondering where she stood on such matters.

Notes

1. In Christopher Moreman's book, *Beyond the Threshold: Afterlife Beliefs and Experiences in World Religions* (Lanham, MD: Rowman & Littlefield, 2017), he outlines in detail the many diverse ways in which the idea of an afterlife is represented and enacted through religious beliefs and practices.
2. Much has been written on the nature of mystical and religious experience. My favorite books include William James, *Varieties of Religious Experience* (New York: Longmans, 1902) and W. T. Stace, *Mysticism and Philosophy* (London: Macmillan, 1961).
3. See S. Stack, J. Gundlach, and J. Reeves, "The heavy metal subculture and suicide," *Suicide and Life-Threatening Behavior* (24:1, 15–23, 1994).
4. S. Freud, *Reflections on War and Death* (New York: Moffat, Yard & Co., 1918) p. 14.
5. E. Benore and C. Park, "Death-specific religious beliefs and bereavement," *International Journal for the Psychology of Religion* (14:1, 1–22, 2004) p. 8.
6. See K. Flannelly et al., "Belief in life after death and mental health," *Journal of Nervous and Mental Disease* (194:7, 524–29, 2006).
7. C. McClain-Jacobson et al., "Belief in an afterlife, spiritual well-being and end-of-life despair in patients with advanced cancer," *General Hospital Psychiatry* (26:6, 484–6, 2004).
8. D. Carr and S. Sharp, "Do afterlife beliefs affect psychological adjustment to late-life spousal loss?" *Journals of Gerontology. Series B, Psychological Sciences and Social Sciences* (69:1, 103–12, 2014) p. 109.

9. K. Hodge, "On imagining the afterlife," *Journal of Cognition and Culture* (11:3/4, 367–89, 2011) pp. 370–71.

10. J. Bering, "Intuitive conceptions of dead agents' minds," *Journal of Cognition and Culture* (2:4, 263–308, 2002) p. 288.

11. V. Pereira, L. Faísca, and R. de Sá-Saraiva, "Immortality of the soul as an intuitive idea," *Journal of Cognition and Culture* (12:1/2, 101–27, 2012) p. 116.

12. R. Bucke, *Cosmic Consciousness* (New York: Dutton & Co., 1923, 1901). Thomas Merton wrote about his fascination with Zen Buddhism late in life in *Zen and the Birds of Appetite* (New York: New Directions, 1968).

13. C. Moreman, in *Beyond the Threshold*, covers many versions of afterlife in world religions including five chapters on Eastern, Islamic, and African traditions.

14. While the range of afterlife narratives are beyond the scope of this book, other writers have explored these, including A. Segal, *Life After Death* (New York: Doubleday, 2010) and Y. Nagasawa and B. Matheson, *The Palgrave Handbook of the Afterlife* (London: Palgrave Macmillan, 2017).

15. The idea of unity in the afterlife is an element in both Hindu and Buddhist traditions and was particularly championed by R. Bucke, *Cosmic Consciousness*.

16. Discussion of biological explanations for near-death experiences, such as drug reactions and brain reactions, can be found in R. Cant et al., "The divided self: Near death experiences of resuscitated patients," *International Emergency Nursing* (20:2, 88–93, 2012).

17. Kenneth Ring, *Life After Death: A Scientific Investigation of the Near-Death Experience* (New York: Coward, McCann and Geoghenan, 1980).

18. A. Sleutjes, A. Moreira-Almeida, and B. Greyson examine 266 publications on near-death experiences in "Almost 40 years investigating near-death experiences," *Journal of Nervous and Mental Disease* (202:11, 833–36, 2014).

19. B. Greyson, "The Near-Death Experience Scale," *Journal of Nervous and Mental Disease* (171:6, 369–75, 1983).

20. For Australia, M. Perera, G. Padmasekara, and J. Belanti, "Prevalence of near-death experiences in Australia," *Journal of Near-Death Studies* (24, 109–16, 2005); for Germany, H. Knoblauch, I. Schmied, and B. Schnettler, "Different kinds of near-death experience";, for the United States, G. Gallup and W. Proctor, *Adventures in Immortality* (New York: McGraw-Hill, 1982).

21. This is summarized by B. Greyson in "Reduced death threat in near-death experiencers," in R. Neimeyer, ed., *Death Anxiety Handbook* (London: Routledge, 2015), pp. 169–80, and is also discussed in relation to resuscitation in hospitals by R. Cant et al., "The divided self."

22. M. Kinsella, "Near-death experiences and networked spirituality," *Journal of the American Academy of Religion* (85:1, 168–98, 2017).

23. Some researchers have argued that what is revealed in near-death experiences should be taken more seriously, including P. Bhattacharya, "Is there science behind the near-death experience?" *Annals of Tropical Medicine and Public Health* (6:2, 151–65, 2013) p. 151, and E. Facco, C. Agrillo, and B. Greyson, "Epistemological implications

of near-death experiences and other non-ordinary mental expressions," *Medical Hypotheses* (85:1, 85–93, 2015).

24. K. Augustine, "Near-death experiences are hallucinations," in M. Martin and K. Augustine, eds., *The Myth of an Afterlife* (Lanham, MD: Rowman & Littlefield, 2015) p. 529.

25. Christian notions of an afterlife are discussed by L. Rudder Baker in, "Death and the afterlife," in W. Wainwright, ed., *The Oxford Hanbook of Philosophy of Religion* (New York: Oxford Univesity Press, 2007) pp. 366–91.

26. R. F. Almeder, *Death and Personal Survival* (Lanham: Rowman & Littlefield, 1992).

27. T. Nichols, *Death and Afterlife* (Grand Rapids, MI: Brazos Press, 2010) p. 13.

28. B. Matheson, "Practical identity," in Y. Nagasawa and B. Matheson, eds., *The Palgrave Handbook of the Afterlife* (pp. 391–411).

29. M. Martin and K. Augustine, eds., *The Myth of an Afterlife*.

30. A. Eschleman, "The afterlife: Beyond belief," *International Journal of the Philosophy of Religion* (80:2, 163–83, 2016).

31. J. Twenge et al., "Declines in American adults' religious participation and beliefs, 1972–2014," *Sage Open* (6:1, 1–13, 2016).

9

Self-Generative Process

The fourth and final enabling frame, self-generative process, is the most neb-
ulous because it draws on various strands of thinking to achieve a radical
shift in perspective. This makes this chapter conceptually challenging because it steps out beyond common ways of thinking and moves into sparsely
mapped and uncertain territory. Despite this, the self-generative frame does
have advantages over its rivals, particularly for those less comfortable with
the more traditional and more theologically oriented options discussed previously. To introduce it briefly, the frame's overarching intent is to position a
relationship with my-death as generated by its own activity. It achieves this
in three important steps: first, it avoids reference to any kind of entity beyond the relationship driving its presence; next, it focuses on the potency
of interconnections between my-death and other aspects of life and their
ability to activate generative processes; and, finally, it engages with the idea
that the reality of this relationship emerges from doing or performing it and
not from independent, external forces. At this stage, these steps might seem
peculiar, but as the chapter proceeds, and, with Brenda providing the focal
point, their meaningfulness will gradually unfold. But before exploring these
ideas, Brenda was facing a quandary regarding her relationship to my-death.

Mandy arrived home from work to find Brenda sitting at the kitchen table
reading a book. "Aren't you on afternoon shifts at the moment?"

"Ah, no. I decided to take two weeks leave," said Brenda as she closed her
book. "Well, actually, it was my supervisor who suggested I take some sick
leave."

"But you don't look sick. What's happened?"

"Um." Brenda looked away.

"Look, you don't really have to tell me anything," said Mandy walking
across to the table. She then sat down and gently touched Brenda's hand.
"I'm just concerned that you're okay."

"No, no, I want to talk . . . I just don't know where to start." Brenda looked
confused. It was normally she who listened to the anguish of others. "It

became obvious I wasn't coping when I walked out of an admission interview a couple days ago. See, I was discussing with the patient how he was
handling his situation, you know, his terminal condition, then, without
warning, I felt totally overwhelmed . . . ah, overwhelmed by the enormity
of what he was facing. I didn't know what to say or how to help him. How
could I help him when I was so confused? I felt like I'd fallen into a dark
hole with no way out."

"That's awful."

"I pride myself on how well I handle strong emotions, and I've never
shied away from discussing tough topics. Sometimes I've cried alongside
patients when they're crying . . . always in an appropriate and controlled
way. . . . But what I was feeling with this patient wasn't appropriate nor was
it controlled; my response was all to do with me and nothing to do with the
patient. I knew I had to leave the interview. So I pretended I needed to go to
the washroom. But then, when I clicked the door of the toilet cubicle, these
uncontrollable waves of strong emotion crashed over me."

"Sadness, grief, anger . . . waves of what?"

"All of those; I didn't really know what was going on." She stared forlornly at the table top. "There'd been some signs earlier in the week something was up. On a couple of mornings I felt a sinking feeling as I went to
work; I didn't really want to go, and that's so unlike me; I'm usually keen to
start the day." She sat in silence trying to think what to say next.

"Brenda, I can't help wondering whether all our talk about death
might've had something to do with it?"

"Yes, I think it has. We all have such different views." She placed her
elbows on the table and cushioned her chin in her hands. "I think I've been
particularly unsettled watching what Stan's going through. I'm feeling very
confused about my views on death. I need to sort it out before I can work
closely with dying patients again."

"So, what's been getting to you?"

"I guess, I've been listening to you, Leo, and Stan explaining your different ways of relating to your own death, but none of them seems right for
me . . . but I'm not sure of an alternative."

Brenda's discussions with the other characters had simulated an interest in
my-death, but she did not find any of their options satisfactory. She needed
to devote time to exploring whether there might be another frame that she
would be happy to inhabit.

Representationism

The three previous enabling frames—structures, suffusion, and transition—have each drawn, in their different ways, on the notion of a some sort of beyond—whether that be a realm or a process or an infrastructural entity—that somehow transcends and makes it possible and meaningful for us to engage in a relationship with my-death. This assumption of a beyond realm is recognized in philosophy as *representationism* (also called "representationalism" or "intentionalism") and is a philosophical position that forms part of a realist theory of knowledge. It argues that our minds process mental images—or representations—of what exists for real outside the mind. It is linked to another aspect of realism, a dualist belief in the separation of the mind from the world. Accordingly, the key task faced in acquiring knowledge is one of finding ways to show whether or not an image or an idea in the mind corresponds to what is actually going on in the world. For a study of my-death, the main challenge would be to show how a particular central idea of my-death is reflected in what is happening somewhere else. But what would happen if the expectations generated by realism and representationism were put to one side? What if we were to see such a relationship as not representing anything?

Brenda had finished tidying up her room and washing the kitchen floors. Now she could relax; ideally relax with other people around. She glanced toward the back of the property and noticed the gap in the fence. She felt it calling and so, with little hesitation, she walked through it and knocked on Stan's door.

"Good, I was just thinking of having a coffee; now, here you are ready to share it with me."

She took up her seat at the kitchen table and watched Stan as he shuffled slowly along the counter, pacing each movement and breaking them into separate tasks, as though he needed to think through each action one at a time. How much slower he's become since going to hospital.

Stan paused and glanced across at Brenda. "We sure have been talking a lot about our mortality lately."

"Yes, that's for sure. It's really forcing me to clarify my views."

"What? I thought those working with the dying would've sorted all that out ages ago?"

"Well, yes, when you're working with it all day, you have much more opportunity than most people to think about death, including your own death."

Stan walked across and placed the mugs of coffee and a plate of chocolate-covered cookies on the table. "So you've managed to clarify things?"

"I suppose we act as though we know death well, patients expect it, but deep down we're just as prone to being confused as anyone else. Some of my colleagues have seen so much death they are almost immune to what they are dealing with; they are good at showing concern and empathy, but deep down I suspect it barely touches them. Kind of a survival strategy, I suppose." She carefully sipped her hot coffee. "Then there's another religious group who rattle on to patients about what happens after death. Others talk to patients but never disclose their own views . . . maybe I fall into that category."

"So, how do you view it?"

"I don't know what to think anymore. I agree with Mandy that life and death need to be seen as a package attached to something else. I can see what she's getting at, but I don't really believe in an afterlife. I think it's all wrapped up together. Sort of self-contained." She gazed out. "I agree with Leo that death is integral to everything, but I don't believe in underlying structures or in manifestations of Being, and all that."

"Okay, so what about my perspective?"

"Yes, yes, I'm getting to that," she said looking directly at Stan. "I get it that my-death is linked to everything that holds me and binds me, everything that makes me finite, and that this can be a constant relationship, but, you too, you're also suggesting this is driven by something else; that finitude and death are two interacting forces operating somewhere behind, above, below, or perhaps even within our experience."

"Yeah, I guess that's the way I see it. How would it be possible otherwise?" He crossed his arms awkwardly. "The way I see it, if you don't refer to the forces within them, then they have no legitimacy; any sense of your own death could be dismissed as a hallucination or as a hiccup in the brain or something. . . . My relationship to death needs to be connected to other forces otherwise it has little meaning."

"But I reckon the experience of relationship to death is real enough in itself; it doesn't need to be linked to anything else."

In Brenda's work with the dying, she had floated flexibly along the various currents of other people's conceptions of my-death. She was able to see the merits of each system and to adjust her language to suit whatever frame her patients preferred: at one moment she could talk about going to heaven, at another she could talk about the power of primordial forces. But in among her ability to move between frames, she had failed to clarify to herself where exactly she stood.

Brenda had also become less comfortable with the idea that my-death could be approached as an image or a signal that pointed to some form of reality that lay beyond how things appeared: a heaven, a God, a primordial force, a fundamental structure, or the like.

Stan stood up from the table and wandered across to the counter to switch on the kettle. "Another coffee?"

"No, I'm okay," said Brenda politely raising her hand in emphasis. "Sounds like you're quite comfortable with some sort of primal impulse driving finitude?"

"Oh, I've always thought that behind everything I experience is another reality. Like the Buddhists say, the everyday world of appearances is an illusion and what is real lies elsewhere."

"But if it lies elsewhere, how can you access it? And if you do access it, how can you know anything about it?"

Stan walked slowly back to the table then sat down and sipped his coffee. "Those are interesting questions. . . . Why do I see things that way?" he asked scratching his chin. "Well, some years ago, in a philosophy night-class, I was introduced to the thinking of the classical philosophers of ancient Greece. I was amazed how two and a half thousand years ago they were saying things that still make sense today." He paused to take several more sips of his coffee. "Have you ever heard of Plato's allegory of the cave?"

"I've heard of Plato but not much more."

"Well, in one of his most famous dialogues, the *Republic*, he has Socrates—who's the central character in his dialogues—describing a situation where a group of prisoners are chained up and can only see a blank wall in front of them. Behind them is a fire which casts shadows of any objects in front of it onto the blank wall. So the prisoners, whose heads are restrained, can only see the shadows moving on the walls; that becomes what they see as real."

"So, we're imprisoned by what we perceive from our senses?"

"Yes, that's it," he said. "Now Plato's idea is that if we could free ourselves from our shackles and could see what was actually going on, then we'd realize the shadows on the wall aren't real in themselves but are representations of another reality."

"Hmm, then the objects making the shadows are more real . . . and I suppose the fire itself is even more real again."

"Yes, that's kind of what he's suggesting. And this is how I see it with death. I'm busy watching the world around me and all that contains and conditions it, but, when I think about it, I see the forces of finitude shaping what goes on and then, when I think more about it, I see the power of my own death driving finitude."

Brenda looked down and stated "I agree with you that death is powerful, personal, and all-pervading but, like Mandy and Leo, this relies on assuming some form of powerful beyond, whether that's a primal impulse or God or Being itself . . . I just don't feel comfortable with accepting any of these. I don't like the idea of my relationship to death being based on something else, something which I have no direct access to. I don't see why my contact with death needs to be seen as representing anything other than itself."

As suggested by Stan's outline of Plato's allegory of the cave, representationism is deeply embedded in traditions of Western thinking from ancient Greece, through medieval Christian theology, onto the European Renaissance, and then reaching its peak in the realism of the Enlightenment with its celebration of empirical science. One example of representationism from this time was the eighteenth-century German philosopher Immanuel Kant whose thinking on the nature and boundaries of knowledge draws heavily on the distinction between how a thing appears to be ("phenomena") and what it is as a thing-in-itself ("noumena"). He claimed that

> though we cannot know these objects as things in themselves, we must yet be in a position at least to think them as things in themselves; otherwise we should be landed in the absurd conclusion that there can be appearance without anything that appears.[1]

So, behind all that appears in our consciousness lies another reality that underpins how we understand the existence of what we are experiencing.

More recently, philosophers such as Michael Tye (2011), John James (2005), and Michael Thau (2002), have energetically defended the assumptions of representationism.[2] For example, Tye (2009) examined several different versions of representationism and the five main arguments for why it makes sense. In his book *Consciousness Revisited* (Tye, 2011) he claimed that

> As I sit here and stare at the intense blue background on the computer screen before me, I undergo a vivid color experience. In so doing, I am conscious of what it is like for me to undergo this experience. And as I reflect on my situation, it seems to me that I could not be radically wrong about the phenomenal character of my experience. Indeed, it seems to me that there is some sense in which I could not be wrong at all about that phenomenal character.[3]

Tye conveys here a confidence in the reality of both how objects are experienced and how we reflect on these experiences. His confidence in the reality of what lies behind how things appear is reflected in many modern thinkers as diverse as Bertrand Russell, John Searle, and even, controversially, Martin Heidegger.[4]

Relational Processes

Brenda was unhappy with the idea that her contact with death was related or made possible because of something else, particularly when that something else lay out of reach of what she could directly experience. The American feminist theorist of science, Karen Barad, has labeled this tendency to image up external sources as "thingafication." She described how

> ... the turning of relations into 'things,' 'entities,' 'relata'—infects much of the way we understand the world and our relationship to it. Why do we think that the existence of relations requires relata? Does the persistent distrust of nature, materiality, and the body that pervades much of contemporary theorizing and a sizable amount of the history of Western thought feed off of this cultural proclivity?[5]

Other thinkers, such as Richard Rorty, Ian Hacking, and Andrew Pickering, have similarly criticized this tendency to automatically assume that linked to each major aspect of our experience lies something separate and real which enables that experience to take place; that behind each representation in our minds lies something on the outside that is being represented.[6] For example, Rorty (2009) argued against what he called "mirror of nature" mentality that contaminates much of Western thinking. He proposed that not all experience is a mirror of another reality and, true to his roots in American pragmatism, stated that we need to look more closely at our social practices.

> *There is nothing deep down inside us except what we have put there ourselves,*
> *no criterion that we have not created in the course of creating a practice, no*
> *standard of rationality that is not an appeal to such a criterion, no rigorous*
> *argumentation that is not obedience to our own conventions.*[7]

Rorty was reacting to our automatic tendency to assume that all objects of our experience are grounded in another source, and Brenda was, similarly, growing increasingly disenchanted with how this played out with my-death.

Late in the afternoon, Mandy strode into her kitchen and hoisted three bags of groceries onto the counter. She glanced over to the table. "Oh, Brenda, there you are, I didn't notice; you're sitting so quietly."

Brenda sat upright at the table staring vacantly out the kitchen window. It looked unusual because she wasn't reading as she normally did and the table was bare.

"How long have you been sitting there?" asked Mandy.

"Maybe an hour or so." With her body in the same position she slowly turned her head to face Mandy. "All week my thoughts have been going round and round trying to figure out how to think about death. It's exhausting, and I'm not getting much sleep."

"Okay, okay," said Mandy taking off her coat and walking across to sit opposite her. She studied Brenda's face and noticed swelling around her eyes. "Just take your time. Tell me some of what's going on."

"It's just that . . . at work I'm focused on other people's death and not ever thinking about my own. And following all our conversations, I don't know what to think anymore."

"Hmm, that must be troubling."

"See," Brenda paused to collect her thoughts, "see, it all started a few weeks ago when I interviewed a women for her first admission into the hospice. She was in her mid-forties and had only recently been diagnosed with a terminal condition. She had two beautiful teenage children, and I remember thinking she was far too young to die." She looked down at the table. "But she seemed different from many others at first admission. She already seemed fairly resigned, even calm with the idea of her approaching death. I was intrigued, so I asked if she believed in an afterlife; she told me she didn't. Then I asked her if she had felt engaged with death earlier in her life; she said yes, she saw death as part and parcel of what it means to be alive. I asked if this was driven by some other force, or presence; perhaps by something in heaven—God, Being, or whatever; she said no, it was sufficient in itself; death doesn't need anything else."

"Hmm, sounds like she's got it figured out."

"I remember finding her last statement, 'death doesn't need anything else,' very curious. I didn't know what she meant. But over the last week my thoughts keep returning to it and thinking about it in different ways."

"Like what?"

"She could have meant, 'you can't think about it any further.' But she would have said that. No, I think she meant death stands on its own, stands for itself. It doesn't need to be propped up with reference to other domains like heaven or primordial forces." Brenda glanced quickly at Mandy. "Sorry, I know that's what you think."

"Don't worry. Go on," Mandy nodded.

"I get what she meant, but I don't have her confidence. I don't know how to think of my death as standing alone, particularly when I'm surrounded by others who seem so confident about it representing something else."

An alternative way of looking at how things might stand by themselves was suggested, ironically, by Immanuel Kant, the same philosopher identified earlier as a champion of representationism. Faced with the primacy of certain concepts, particularly as they relate to the foundations of ethics, in a small corner of his vast thinking, Kant proposed what he called the three "postulates of practical reason" which he applied to God, immortality, and freedom.[8] While knowledge and reason do not give us direct access to these concepts, he suggested that they are postulated in the process of living an ethical life. He saw it as more than living as if God, immortality, and freedom existed; the act of living is undertaken with these as a base; they are posited through the process of engagement and in this way they become real—not real in the sense of solid rocks or houses, but real in the sense of love and injustice. By assuming and absorbing them into the way we live our lives, they become real in the process. For example, it is difficult to justify our belief in free will when so much of our behavior is controlled by other factors such as genetics, culture, and social context. But since we act constantly *as though* we are free, freedom becomes posited in our actions and in this way becomes, for all intents and purposes, real in our lives. Now, Kant's postulates have been heavily criticized because acting *as though* freedom is real is not the same thing as actually being real, but the idea does open up some interesting possibilities.[9]

Half a century later another German philosopher, G. W. H. Hegel, was grappling with similar dilemmas in his exploration of the reality of appearances.[10] While, like Kant, much of his thinking leaned toward representationism, when he came to consider the nature of how things appeared in our experience, he, unlike Kant, avoided positing a realm behind appearances which enabled them to happen. He claimed

> *[that] the reflection-in-another of what exists concretely is, however, not separate from the reflection-in-itself; the ground is their unity, from which the concrete existence has gone forth. What exists thus concretely contains in itself relationality and its multiple connection with other entities existing concretely. Thus, too, it is reflected in itself as ground. As such, what exists concretely is a thing.[11]*

Hegel was pushing the idea that nothing resides behind or beyond the "thing" we see. Its appearance can be considered an unfolding reality in its own right. Its reality emerges from the interconnections between things, not from some other transcendent source.

A further half-century or more on, philosophers such as Alfred North Whitehead (1929) and Charles Hartshorne (1953) were similarly exploring the potential of processes that rely on the dynamic interconnections between things.[12] This echoes the discussion in Chapter 5 on the merits of shifting away from an individualistic approach to identity and toward seeing it in terms of relationships. Relationships are dynamic and ever-changing; each relationship connects with other relationships, and their multiple links together form into systems. Each individual point in a system of relationships links relationally to this system as a whole, and since this system is constantly changing and constantly becoming something else, each point in this system derives its reality from its part in the whole. As claimed by Whitehead (1938),

> *[a] single fact in isolation is the primary myth required for finite thought, that is to say, for thought unable to embrace totality.*
> *This mythological character arises because there is no such fact. Connectedness is of the essence of all things of all types. It is of the essence*

of types, that they be connected. Abstraction from connectedness involves the omission of an essential factor in the fact considered. No fact is merely itself.[13]

For Whitehead and other process philosophers, reality emerges in the midst of the complex interrelationships between individuals and systems; in the dynamic interplay of part-to-part and of part-to-whole. This they viewed as sufficient in itself, and any appeal to another reality is rendered unnecessary.

So, what does this mean for how we might understand engaging in a relationship to my-death? Could this relationship be viewed as a self-contained process in its own right?

It was four days later, while Brenda and Mandy were sitting facing each other at the kitchen table again, when Mandy asked, "Are you making any progress?"

"Yes, I think I'm moving forward." Brenda smiled then sighed. "But I'm still very confused. . . . What I am sure about is that my relationship to death doesn't need to be based on any connection to a beyond or any other transcendent realm."

"Then, how can you explain the reality of this relationship? I mean, you could just be deluded or hallucinating."

"I kind of know it a bit from my work. Whenever I get in touch with a sense of my own death, it feels so inward; it's totally inward. I sense it has no reference beyond itself other than the way it connects into my life."

"I don't follow. How can it be both inward and connected?"

"No, I mean, not connected to a beyond or to some underlying structures." She glanced down and noticed how tightly she was grasping the side of the table. She relaxed her grip. "What makes it real is the way it is connected to everything else. But not connected like wiring in a house, more connected in a constantly changing and dynamic way. And, since my life is constantly changing, so these connections with death keep changing, and it's within this process, in the dynamics of this constant change, that my relationship with death emerges as real."

Mandy sat back with a confused expression on her face. "I'm sorry. That's a lot to take in." She paused to consider it further. "Actually, I don't really get what you're saying. . . . I don't see anything wrong with accepting a beyond; something behind appearances that makes things possible, like a divine realm or heaven or something."

"Okay, I know it's hard to get your head around, and I'm still working on it." Brenda paused to collect her thoughts. "Let's go back to the concept of finitude. My life is constantly constrained in thousands of ways, little ways and big ways, and I recognize this because I'm in touch with the ways these limitations are signaled or marked. But these constraints and their finitude markers don't occur on their own; rather, they each connect to each other in a constantly changing and dynamic manner. See, it's these connections that provide the energy and force to make my mortality real."

The enabling frame which is beginning to take shape in Brenda's head draws on a different conception of finitude. Each point of contact with finitude—achieved via finitude markers—connects with other points of contact, and together these coalesce into a dynamic system of interconnections in the midst of which a relationship with my-death emerges.

Performative Reality

The English philosopher John L. Austin (1970) introduced an important distinction in the way we use language.[14] First, we use language in ways that conform to representationism, where what we say represents something that is really happening in the outside world and that can be verified as true or false. If someone were to declare, "The cat is caught up the pear tree," then the presence of the cat and the pear tree can be verified by looking up at the tree, and the status of the cat's "caught" relationship can be checked out. But Austin described a second class of statements that he named "performative utterances" and which are not primarily said by way of referencing something out there in the real world and should not, because of that, be evaluated in terms of being either true or false.[15] Instead these statements function alongside the doing of something; they form part of the various things we do with words, such as someone making a promise, or a referee calling a player offside, or a judge passing a sentence. For example, when the bride and groom at a wedding state, "I do," the words do something, they transform each speaker from an unmarried into a married state. Such a statement is neither true nor false, and it is not referencing other sets of relations other than itself. Subsequent writing by Austin and others have identified a range of explicit and implicit performatives, as well as those that can be transformative, and they have illustrated how widely we use language in this way.[16]

Austin's distinction raises questions regarding whether statements about my-death are best seen as representational or performative. What is happening in language when we say, "I am in a relationship with my own death"? Those favoring the three earlier enabling frames would interpret this statement as representational, in that my-death is seen as representing some other supernormal reality. But what happens if we were to consider this as a performative statement, as a statement that is part of the doing of something?

Leo took a break from his study and found Brenda in the living room with her legs curled up on the couch reading a book.

Leo flopped into the armchair. "Hi, what ya reading?"

"It's a book recommended by a nursing colleague. She thought I'd be interested." Brenda turned the book over to look at the cover. "It's called *Gender Trouble*, and it's by this queer feminist writer Judith Butler who...."

"Hmm, interesting. Well, what do you think?"

"I thought it was a bit strange at first, but not so much now I've nearly finished it. It's about how gender is performed as a social and cultural event rather than something hardwired into our biology or our minds. I don't know if my colleague had this in mind—probably not—but I'm finding it very relevant to my challenges with finding a way to think about my own death."

"Okay, okay," stammered Leo, unable to conceal his curiosity. "Tell me more."

"Well, Butler argues that gender shouldn't be viewed as an attribute or essential characteristic of who we are. She describes how we *do* gender, we *perform* it, and it is in the action of performance that it becomes real. I don't identify as a heterosexual woman because of some essential femininity; I identify as such because that is how I live and breathe in all my actions and all my relationships."

"Interesting idea. But how would it play out for you in your life?"

"Ah, a lot of it is revealed in how we use language. See, she makes a distinction between when we are making factual claims about the world that are either true or false and when we are speaking as part of what we do. So if a midwife in the birthing room was to say, 'It's a girl,' this is, at one level, a statement of fact, but it is far more than that. More importantly this initiates all the social expectations of being female that will constitute who that baby is as a woman for the rest of her life."

"I see, so she's saying that many of the ways we speak kind of enact how we intend to be, or, at least, how society intends us to be." Leo glanced across, looking unsure about what he'd just said. "But how does all this stuff on gender relate to death?"

"Ah, okay. As I've told you before, I don't think of my death as a reflecting another reality. I see it as real in its own right." She paused to think over an example. "So, using Judith Butler, when I say something like 'I am going to die,' the main thing I'm highlighting is an action in my life; if you like, I'm doing my relationship with death."

"But you can check out whether that is either true or false."

"No, no; that's where you're wrong. It's impossible for me to check it out because I would need to be dead, and, as you continually point out, my death is total nothingness." Brenda smiled, unfolded her legs and placed the book on the coffee table. "So when I say 'I am going to die,' I'm not intending to describe a state of affairs; more that, in the process of saying it, I'm generating a relationship. It's a performative statement which, by saying it, I locate myself in the midst of something I'm doing all the time."

Judith Butler's influential writing on performativity described the doing of gender as "that reiterative power of discourse to produce the phenomena that it regulates and constrains."[17] Her thinking combined the positions already discussed: a move away from essentialized structures, a focus on the power of relational processes, and an interest in the reality-generating capacity of doing and performing. She managed to weave these positions into a dynamic understanding of reality that has found applications in diverse areas such as gender fluidity, video art, and management studies.

Brenda applied Butler's ideas imaginatively to how she thought about her relationship to my-death. This helped her resolve her dissatisfaction with frames that assume the ontological reality of some form of hidden transcendence. Instead, she moved to seeing my-death as integral to the arena of action in her life; an expanded performance in which my-death permeated all around her. Life and death then became like two interlocked characters in a play; if I can't perform one, I can't perform the other, and vice versa. In the process of acting, something else is simultaneously produced which then extends beyond itself.[18]

"So, Brenda, what does . . ." Leo stretched himself in the armchair then allowed his trunk to slide down to a seated position on the floor. "What does this idea of performing a relationship with death actually mean in how we might live our lives?"

"Look, it's very early days for me to think this way. I'm not sure where it's heading . . . but I'm certainly a lot more comfortable with it than with other ideas."

"Ah ha, 'comfortable' in what way?"

"What I'm trying to say is, in the act of engaging in a relationship with my own death, it posits itself, and I don't need to refer to anything else other than the relationship itself. See, like Judith Butler says, it's in the act of doing or performing the relationship that it comes into being. All I need to do is turn and face it and embrace it and make it part of my life, and through this its reality comes from itself."

"Mmm, but it sounds like she was talking more about social realities; gender, sexuality, social norms, and so on."

"Yes, she is writing in a different domain. But she is fighting some of the same fights: she and I both want to move away from assuming some primordial independent super-reality; we are both shying away from looking at gender or death as representing something else; we both see the power of processes and of interconnections in driving the reality of things, and we see the doing of relationships, the performing of what we are, as vital to what we understand as real."[19]

"All right, I see the parallels.   But I'm not convinced that perceiving yourself in a relationship is the same as actually being in a relationship."

"This is where Stan's talk about the concept of finitude comes in. I am constantly surrounded by signals of my boundedness, or markers of finitude as Stan calls them. Each time I respond to these markers by sensing them, feeling them, or thinking about them, they coalesce as small parts of in a much bigger relationship I have with my own death. So, because of the bountiful availability of finitude markers, I am able, at all times, to access and enact an incremental part of my relationship with death, and these small parts accumulate, like tributaries feeding into a big river, into a much more tangible and meaningful relationship to my death." She glanced across at Leo, who nodded back, then continued, "I guess it's an issue of critical mass. By constantly engaging with finitude I am enacting little bits of what gathers into a more substantial relationship, and it's the constant repetition which makes it real; more real, eventually, than many other things I experience."

Brenda comes back time and time again to seeing reality as cumulatively actualized in performance. On the one hand, my-death is not real because there is nowhere in our lives to point to, but, on the other hand, it is real in the sense of being enacted as a postulate that draws on the many strands of our daily connections with finitude.

This chapter has introduced the fourth of the enabling frames for use in engaging in a relationship with my-death. It began with Brenda's distress at conversations with the dying which had highlighted her not knowing the basis for how she viewed my-death. She then traversed several schools of thought as divergent as American pragmatism, German idealism, and post-modern feminism. While these academic traditions differ in many respects, she saw their interests as converging on a rejection of representationism and a recognition of the power of interconnecting processes to generate their own reality. She then proceeded forward to look at the reality of a relationship with my-death as grounded in repeated daily interaction with finitude. It is in engagement with, or the doing of finitude, that spaces open up for performing a relationship with my-death. This was where she had now arrived, and she was pleased to have found a place where she could feel comfortable. But she also knew that many challenges lay ahead, and she needed to find some way of integrating this perspective into her life.

Notes

1. I. Kant, *Critique of Pure Reason* (Cambridge: Cambridge University Press, 1998) p. Bxxvi. More on Kant's representationism is covered by A. Dickerson, *Kant on Representation and Objectivity* (Cambridge: Cambridge University Press, 2004).
2. J. John, "Representationism, phenomenism, and the intuitive view," *Philosophical Topics* (33:1, 159–84, 2005), and M. Tye, "Representationalist theories of consciousness," in A. Beckermann et al., eds., *The Oxford Handbook of Philosophy of Mind* (New York: Oxford University Press, 2009) pp. 253–67, and M. Thau, *Consciousness and Cognition* (New York: Oxford University Press, 2002).
3. M. Tye, *Consciousness Revisited* (Cambridge, MA: MIT Press, 2011) p. 183.
4. T. Rockmore argues that Heidegger's philosophy is representationist in "Heidegger and representationalism," *History of Philosophy Quarterly* (13:3, 363–74, 1996), whereas W. Blattner argues that Heidegger does not see all experience as representational in "Is Heidegger a representationalist?," *Philosophical Topics* (27:2, 179–204, 1999).
5. K. Barad, "Posthumanist performativity," *Signs: Journal of Women in Culture and Society* (28:3, 810–31, 2003) p. 812.

6. I. Hacking, *Representing and Intervening* (Cambridge: Cambridge University Press, 1983).

7. R. Rorty, *Consequences of Pragmatism* (Minneapolis: University of Minnesota Press, 1991) p. xlii.

8. I. Kant, *Critique of Practical Reason* (Cambridge: Cambridge University Press, 1997, 1788).

9. For example, J. Macintosh heavily criticizes this in "The impossibility of Kantian immortality," *Dialogue* (19:2, 219–234, 1980), whereas S. Gardner identifies some of their potential in "Kant's practical postulates and the limits of the critical system," *Hegel Bulletin* (32:1/2, 187–215, 2013).

10. Hegel discusses many of these ideas in *Phenomenology of Spirit* (Oxford: Oxford University Press, 1977).

11. Hegel *Encyclopedia* (Cambridge: Cambridge University Press, 2010) section 124, pp. 191–92.

12. See A. N. Whitehead, *Process and Reality* (New York: Free Press, 2010) and C. Hartshorne, *Reality as Social Process* (New York: Free Press, 1953). There are many other thinkers with a similar distaste for representationism, including works by notable thinkers such as Henri Bergson, William James, Joseph Rouse, and even Gilles Deleuze.

13. A. N. Whitehead, *Modes of Thought* (New York: Free Press, 1968) p. 9.

14. J. L. Austin, *How to Do Things with Words* (Cambridge, MA: Harvard University Press, 1975).

15. Austin later dealt with these under the title of "illocutionary acts."

16. For example, these have been explored by E. Sedgwick and A. Frank in *Touching Feeling: Affect, Pedagogy, Performativity* (Durham, NC: Duke University Press, 2003).

17. J. Butler, *Bodies That Matter: On the Discursive Limits of Sex* (New York: Psychology Press, 1993) p. 2.

18. Performative ontology has found many uses, including in economics and management theory. For an overview, see J. Loxley, *Performativity* (London: Routledge, 2006).

19. Interestingly, Hegel was a strong formative influence on Butler, and her emphasis on the power of relational processes is likely to have been influenced by his ideas. For example, see her *Subjects of Desire: Hegelian Reflections in Twentieth-Century France* (New York: Columbia University Press, 2012).

10

Dialogue

This book is exploring ways to maintain a lifelong relationship to one's own death. The first two chapters clarified what is meant by my-death by distinguishing it from the death of others (other-death) and from the process of dying. Chapter 3 confronted the problem of my-death lying beyond the bounds of intelligibility; in other words, in contrast to other aspects of life, my-death is essentially an unthinkable and an unspeakable, and perhaps an impossible, possibility. Chapter 4 backed this up by highlighting how this unthinkability contributes to widespread reluctance to contemplate or discuss my-death. In response to this, Chapter 5 then proposed that a lifelong relationship to my-death might be possible through the use of what were described as four enabling frames. These frames—structures, suffusion, transition, and process—provided the focus for each of the next four chapters and were seen, in their own way, as offering accessible touchstones for us to consider ourselves engaging a relationship with my-death. At one level they might be thought of as convenient fictions because they cannot possibly get around the fundamental unthinkability of my-death, but, at another level, once we fully embrace any one of these frames, it offers a focal point for us to at least experience ourselves participating in a relationship with my-death.

This chapter compares the relative strengths and weaknesses of these enabling frames. Other enabling frames are possible, and the ones chosen here could be described in other ways, but, for the purposes of demonstrating the possibilities of ongoing relationships with my-death, discussion will remain focused on these four frames.

Stan placed his suit for special occasions on the bed. This was the suit he wore for weddings and funerals; well, mostly funerals; the last wedding he attended was eight years ago; he's attended maybe six or seven funerals in the last year. It's probably more fitting to call it his funeral suit.

He chose a tie; something bright and suitable for this "special dinner" as Mandy called it. A week ago she had invited him over to celebrate his return to health. He had been struck by the thoughtfulness of her invitation. He felt, indeed, it was the right time to celebrate.

He thought back on the events of the past months: how Leo's curiosity about death had set him thinking, how conversations with Brenda had kindled further interest, how his heart attack had brutally shaken the stability of his daily life, how his months of recuperation had given him time to re-evaluate his relationship to death.

He glanced across at Winston who was watching him from the door. "I'm sorry boy, I think this dinner is too fancy for a dog like you. Can't have you dribbling over everyone."

He sat on the bed and awkwardly pulled up his trousers then buttoned up his white shirt and grappled with knotting his tie. He carefully donned his jacket, flicked a few bits of fluff off the sleeve, then, standing back, he admired his neat appearance in the mirror.

He wondered, with some excitement, what they would end up talking about over dinner.

Poles Apart

How might we compare these four very different ways of engaging with my-death? Each involved different and separate traditions of thinking, with many places at which their ideas clashed.

Stan drew in a sharp breath as he walked through from Mandy's kitchen into the dining room. A host of flickering candles had been placed around the room and on each available surface stood bunches of flowers in vases. In pride of place, in the center of the table, the largest vase of all was holding a host of long-stemmed sunflowers. He loved sunflowers, their bright beaming faces welcoming everyone around them.

Brenda and Mandy were busy walking back and forth from the kitchen with utensils and dishes. They were both wearing stylish long dresses with their tops adorned in jewelry. Leo was already sitting at the table. He was wearing neat trousers and a formal white shirt, but he couldn't bring himself to wear a tie.

When everything was out on the table, they all sat down and Brenda poured bubbly wine into tall glasses.

With ceremonial propriety, Mandy raised her glass and the others followed. "I want to toast Stan's recovery. It's been a hard few months, but now he's back and fully independent . . . a little slower, but a captain in charge of his own ship."

The others raised their glasses. "To Stan."

Mandy smiled warmly at each of the others as they sipped their wine. "I know he's recovered because yesterday I saw him planting his tomatoes." She looked directly at Stan. "I also want to take this opportunity to acknowledge his contribution to our lives. All four of us have been on a journey; an unusual journey, but one that has helped us in connecting to our own deaths. And, for me, it was Stan who helped me move forward."

"Yes, we've all had so many conversations on the topic," Stan agreed. "But really it was your own doing. In fact, it was Leo's curious questioning that started me off. He's the one who set the ball rolling. I was just there to listen and merely joined in with my own stuff when. . . ."

" . . . I tell you what," interrupted Leo, "since we're all together, why don't we each take turns to describe where we've got to. I think we've done this one-to-one with each other, but never all together. Let's see where it takes us?"

"Without arguing, you mean?" queried Brenda.

"I'm not sure. Let's try to avoid shouting and put downs, but it's okay to disagree. Come on, let's see where it leads."

Since they have each adopted radically different platforms for interacting with my-death, one would naturally expect this initial discussion to focus on points of disagreement. Despite the friendly occasion, Leo's suggestion was undoubtedly risky since their marked differences in views could lead discussion to deteriorate into hostile argument. So let's see how they handle these main areas of disagreement.

The first major point of contention between the frames concerned the issue of continuity. Does my-death mark a final endpoint, or is it a point of transition from one form of life to another?

Mandy helped Leo bring out their entrée: scallops in cream sauce, his first attempt at such fancy cooking.

After everyone had tasted their portion and praised Leo for his contribution, he raised his hands to signal he wanted to say something. "Okay, okay. Since I apparently started this all off, I'll go first. Now, you've heard this from me many times before, but I'll say it again: my death is final. When I die, my consciousness will cease to function, which means, from my point of view, everything will cease to exist: I go, my consciousness goes, the whole world ceases to be . . . total annihilation. This is because my death is integral and an essential condition for me being alive. This is all we can say about it."

"As we've already discussed, I don't see death as final," stated Mandy emphatically, taking another sip of wine. "I'm totally convinced that after I die my life will continue in some form. I must admit I'm not quite sure what form it will take because I won't be able to test it out until I die, but everything around suggests to me that this is what will happen."

"Oh, but Mom, your solution, the fairy tale of an afterlife, it simply makes no sense. Also, if you've no idea what form it will take, why do you need it? It's totally unnecessary."

"Hold on, young man," interrupted Stan detecting some hostility in Leo's voice. "Your mother is just as entitled as you to think of death in the way she's choosing. I'm not as sure of the existence of an afterlife as her, but I have no reason to count it out. I'd say it's just as rational as you viewing your death as the end of everything, except it allows us to think about it in a more relaxed way. What do you think, Brenda?"

"Hmm," responded Brenda as she thoughtfully chewed her last scallop. "On this issue, I'm with Leo." She put down her fork and glanced across at Mandy. "I'm sorry; while I can understand the advantages of an afterlife, I don't think I need it for the purposes of my relationship to death. I think death is just there as it is; actually, it's everywhere but nowhere beyond itself."

Leo and Mandy have occupied polar opposite positions on the issue of continuity. If restricted to their views, we would be faced with choosing between one of only two possible positions. Stan and Brenda both introduced in-between positions where, for Stan, an afterlife seemed equally possible as looking at it as a total end, and where, for Brenda, an afterlife was retransposed into the present. This suggests that instead of looking at this tension as involving an all-or-nothing binary, it could be approached as continuum along which there are a spectrum of different possibilities.

The second main area of contention concerned whether my-death is best thought of as a structural condition for the possibility of life or whether it is something that permeates all aspects of one's finite being.

Stan turned to Leo sitting beside him. "Leo, I'd like to pick up on your idea of death as a necessary condition for what it means to exist. I've done some thinking about this, and, I must say, when I look at death this way it does seem to make sense; death seems to be integral to what it means to be alive. But then, when I take it further, when I think about how we understand structuring principles in other contexts, say with structure in a building or structure in the composition of matter, then this way of looking at things appears more and more like a metaphor than an accurate and literal depiction of what's going on." Stan glanced at Brenda then Mandy, then back at Leo. "As far as I'm concerned, I see death *as though* it's part of the structure of existence, but, as with all metaphors, this is, in effect, a simpler way of understanding an aspect of something that is far more complex."

Leo emptied his glass of wine. "So, you're saying my view isn't pointing toward anything accurate or real; it's just a convenient comparison that bears little relationship to what is going on in the real world."

"No, no. I'm saying it seems real when your mind is held by it, but you aren't constrained by it. I can shift into another way of looking at it, another metaphor, which can seem just as real as soon as I buy into it."

"So its realness is illusory?"

"What does illusion mean here?" queried Stan with a warm grin spreading across his face. "Each of us has agreed at some point that mortality isn't directly knowable or thinkable, which means we need to turn to indirect ways of talking about it. These aren't illusions; they are for each of us our own best approximations."

"What you're suggesting," joined in Brenda, "could apply to all our approaches to death. We're making use of different metaphors, different ways of looking *as if* mortality is like something else."

"Yes," said Stan. "Which means that several possibilities can coexist at the same time. You can choose which orientation you want to make real. For example, and apologies to you Leo, I find the metaphor of a conditioning structure somewhat static and impersonal. The metaphor I favor is one of like an electrical surge through the body. When I connect with finitude, when I see finitude as a force penetrating everywhere, I feel totally immersed in my mortality in an emotionally charged way."

The figurative use of language in relation to death, particularly in the form of metaphor, has attracted some interest. For example, James Sexton (1997) analyzed the variety of metaphors used by medical clinicians in talking about the death and dying of their patients. Common examples included sleep metaphors—"put to rest"—leaving metaphors—"he's gone"—and loss metaphors—"sorry about your loss."[1] Bob Spall and colleagues (2001) invited thirty-one end-of-life professionals to talk about death in small focus groups and then analyzed their use of metaphors and, subsequently, found a rich variety of categories including traveling metaphors—"climbing a mountain"—endpoint metaphors—"coming to a full stop"—and environment metaphors—"being in a fog."[2] However, these and other studies on death have primarily focused on the use of metaphors in talking about other-death and the process of dying, not on their use in talking about my-death. Larence Ross and Howard Polio (1991), in one of the few studies I found on metaphors and my-death, analyzed how twenty-six Americans talked about it and found that metaphors helped convey negativity, ambivalence, and positivity in how they related to my-death.[3] But, despite Stan's insistence on the importance of metaphor, research on their use in talking about my-death remains still relatively unexplored.

The third main area of contention concerns whether or not a relationship with my-death requires assuming the existence of an external source or a transcendental platform as part of an enabling frame.

Brenda was sitting forward, sipping her wine and nibbling from a bowl of nuts. "Okay, this is what I find difficult with how you three are approaching death. It seems to me each of you is assuming death is connected with something that exists, either behind or beyond it, that enables it to act as a force in our lives. Mandy, you talk about heaven as a place for a continuing afterlife; and Stan, well, your emotional embrace of finitude and death seems to me to rely on posing some form primordial force operating behind both. And Leo. . . ."

"Well, my approach doesn't make any such assumptions," interrupted Leo. "I don't claim there's anything beyond death except nothingness."

"Leo, I agree with you, there will be no afterlife after I die. I was brought up to believe in God and to see his power holding creation together and ensuring our place in his heavenly realm after we die. But this God ceased to mean anything to me long ago. And, in my book, without God, there can be no heaven and no life after death."

"I find that such a pointless and depressing view," commented Mandy.

"Hmm," said Leo as he poured himself another glass of bubbly. "I managed to escape Sunday school, sermons, church ceremonies, and all that; I guess that's why I never took the idea of God that seriously."

"So, Leo," continued Brenda, "like you, I think of my death as a blank nothingness . . . but I realize I can't even say that because the idea of nothingness draws on the idea of a continuing somethingness, and that's certainly not what I mean." She paused. "However, unlike you, I don't see my life here as grounded in anything else."

"But that's not what I'm saying," said Leo in a tone betraying his annoyance.

"Ah, but . . . ," broke in Stan, "how can my death have any meaning if it isn't backed up by something else? To mean something, it needs to refer to something."

Brenda turned her gaze between each of the speakers. "I think there is a way, by. . . ."

"So if nothing happens after death," interrupted Mandy, "then you can't form any form of legacy; it's pointless building empires, raising children, completing fine art works; none of these matter?"

"Okay, okay, hold up all of you," said Brenda raising her voice and beginning to wonder whether they'd drunk too much wine. "I can't respond to all your arguments at once. Let's just calm down and deal with them one at a time." She paused, then resumed in a lower and a calmer tone. "Leo, I agree, you're not saying something persists in time after death, but you are still assuming a beyond; not a beyond in time, but a beyond in terms of an underlying structure; you know, this unifying function of Being that you talk about that holds everything together."

"Hmm," replied Leo taking another sip of wine.

"And, Mandy," continued Brenda, "without an afterlife, it doesn't matter what happens after you die, so your legacy isn't in itself of much importance. It matters only insofar as it's relevant to what you see as valuable and meaningful in the present. What really matters is what I do here and now. I can't bank on anything beyond. I need to focus on living the best life I can: hurting as few people as possible, forming close and loving relationships, engaging in life as well as I can; but not engaging with it in terms of a life beyond my death."

"So protecting the planet and educating your children are pointless?" queried Mandy.

"They do matter in so much as they relate to the meaning of what is happening now, but not in terms of what will happen after I die."

"Okay," joined in Stan, "so what does it matter whether or not you live a meaningful or a good life? If there's no reference point beyond yourself, then surely it's all arbitrary. Whether you live a meaningful or pointless life makes no difference. So why bother?"

Brenda switched her glance between each of her adversaries. She felt their combined challenges were pushing her into a corner. She wanted their conversation to return to a more even dialogue. "Why don't we see about the main course?"

For Brenda, her self-generative process frame allowed her to avoid assuming a separate, unobservable reality acting as a powerhouse for what my-death represented. She felt uncomfortable conjuring up alternative, hidden realms with only tentative links to everyday life. For the other three, the idea of separate realities was already well embedded into their thinking, embedded to an extent that they struggled to see it otherwise. Moreover, each of these other realities also played a crucial role as reference points grounding other key aspects of existence which included a foundation for determining what was virtuous and ethical and a means by which to connect with deceased lovedones. Their challenges forced her to realize that she had little chance of persuading them to engage in considering the merits of her frame.

Common Ground

Despite these points of difference and potential disagreement, our four diners also shared views on some common advantages in engaging with each of their respective enabling frames. The first positive feature concerned the prospect of entering into a more meaningful relationship with my-death.

Mandy walked out of the kitchen with the main course, veal cordon bleu. She had worked hard that afternoon wrapping the veal slices in ham and cheese and layering them with a batter and preparing a rich sauce. It seemed a special enough recipe for this special occasion. Brenda and Leo followed her out ferrying platters of roasted potatoes, cooked vegetables, and two bowls of salad.

Stan rubbed his hands in delight. "This looks wonderful. Truly out-standing." He opened a bottle of red wine and poured a small amount into each of their second glasses.

After everyone was seated, Mandy suggested, "So far, we've been talking about the differences between our approaches to death; now, instead, why don't we turn this around and look at what we have in common, look at what we agree on?"

"Hmm, I'd support that," responded Brenda looking up at the ceiling and pausing to consider her position. "Well, the first thing that strikes me is how we've all agreed that forming an ongoing relationship to death is worthwhile."

Leo was quick to concur. "Yes. Before I didn't even see it as a subject worth thinking about. Now, having thought about it, having *really* thought about it, it's opened up a whole new world of ideas. I never thought death would connect with so many different philosophies."

"Surprisingly," said Stan directing a wry smile at Leo, "despite our age difference, it's fairly similar for me. Perhaps I'm a bit slow off the mark be-cause, before my heart attack, I didn't think about it much and probably avoided it at times. This all changed when death reached out and touched me. Now, thanks in no small measure to our conversations, I find myself perfectly relaxed in talking about my own death."

Mandy swallowed a mouthful of cordon bleu then declared, "And for me, I've spent too much time and energy running away from death; ducking and diving, and avoiding any thoughts about it. I saw it as negative and morbid, and I didn't really want a relationship with it. How silly is that?" She smiled across at Leo. "Ever since my encounter with the certainty of an afterlife, I now find I'm quite relaxed about it; I'm happy to relate to it."

Brenda spooned some beans onto her plate. "What I like about the way all of us have managed to establish relationships to death is that we've done it together. Our journeys have brought us together. We have each, in our own way, found some footing upon which to connect, and connect mean-ingfully, with each other."

During the course of this book, the four characters have successfully nego-tiated pathways through my-death's fog of unintelligibility to discover their own basis for entering a relationship with my-death. While settling on dif-ferent frames, the sequence was remarkably similar. At first my-death lurked in the background, a topic either of little significance or too threatening to contemplate, then some form of critical incident drew it into the foreground: for Leo, it was his sensitive response at Aunty Sue's funeral; for Stan, it was his heart attack; for Mandy, it was her mystical experience; and for Brenda, it was a crisis at work. Then, in the context of open discussion, they clarified the central idea of a new frame of reference which they further developed and reinforced through more discussion. Confidence in their frame then slowly consolidated to a point where they felt my-death had become a regular part of daily living.

The next common feature concerned the way their respective enabling frames have helped them speak about my-death.

Stan munched his last piece of chicken, placed his knife and fork down, then used his napkin to swipe across his smiling lips. "You know, a few months ago we couldn't have had this conversation."

"One of us might have tried," said Brenda, "but we would've ended up in an awkward silence."

"In the past," continued Stan, "in moments when I'm likely to think about mortality, say at a funeral or in a hospital, I'd start to think about it, then feel confused, then feel a little bit scared, then I'd snap myself out of it by thinking about other things."

"Yeah, that's because you really didn't have a way of thinking about it," observed Leo.

Stan nodded his agreement. "So, while our approaches differ, they have allowed us to think more about death, and, because of this, we're also more likely to talk about it . . . even though we speak in slightly different languages."

"I think it's a confidence thing," suggested Mandy. "I no longer feel threatened because I'm confident about the way I see things. What you others think is your business; I'm not going to try to convince you otherwise." She sipped some red wine. "But it just helps to know that each of you has managed to connect with death and kind of understands what I'm getting at."

"Yes, that's right," said Brenda, "but it's also about being clear of the difference between my death and other people's death. Since I'm surrounded with death at work, I thought I was familiar with my own death, but I now realize I was mostly connecting to the death of other people. I spent most my time talking about their deaths and seldom talking about my own. When we started talking together—mostly driven by you, Leo, I might add—I was surprised to find it quite difficult at first; difficult, I guess, because it highlighted how little I'd actually thought about it."

The companions attribute their confidence in talking about my-death to, first, discovering a frame that enabled them to form a relationship with my-death, then to having time to consolidate their trust in that frame, and, finally, to recognizing it in other people which then provided them with a basis for meaningful conversations. The interesting point Stan added was that perhaps the nature of a frame mattered less than the act of engaging with it. People could engage with a whole array of different frames, but what counts is how the frame they chose facilitates their conversations about my-death. Which frame suits which person is up to them to explore and decide; what matters is how the adopted frame makes it possible to jump over the unspeakable nothingness of my-death and engage with it as a continuous relationship.

A final common feature to crop up in their conversation concerned the way finitude played a part in their contact with my-death.

Stan turned in his seat to face Leo. "Now, young man, it was you who first introduced me to Heidegger's concept of finitude, and ever since I've been thinking about it and developing it in my own way.[4] I now see finitude as permeating every aspect of my bounded existence, and I am reminded of this through the many signals or finitude markers that constantly surround me."

"Thanks, Stan," said Leo, "but you seemed to have taken it down quite a different path than what I was intending."

"I know, but Heidegger wasn't the only thinker in this area." He turned his seat back to its original position. "There's one aspect of finitude he didn't really explore and that's its relationship to suffering. See, suffering crops up in many parts of our lives and on many occasions. Suffering constrains what we do, and, what's more, the prospect of suffering plays a key role in our worries about dying."[5]

Mandy was staring vaguely at the sunflowers. "Stan, I found your take on finitude very interesting . . . particularly when I was grappling with the meaning of my mystical encounter. It was these finitude markers that put me in touch with death and constantly alerted me to it as the gateway to eternal life. As you say, the markers are everywhere, and they serve to constantly remind me of the certainty of an afterlife."

"Hmm, finitude markers," muttered Brenda, feeling a little light-headed from the wine. "They help keep me in touch with my death. Although I don't see them as marking or signaling something else; rather, they mark the way death is constantly enacting itself in my continuing existence." She paused, recognizing she was in the process of adjusting to her new frame and was still working out ways to talk about it.

Leo looked across at Brenda and nodded his understanding. "Well, it didn't start this way but somehow all four of us have managed to include finitude markers as active in maintaining contact with our own deaths. It doesn't seem to matter much what interpretation of mortality we take on, we all use these markers as a contact point for sustaining our awareness of death."

"But would we have accessed our various perspectives without these markers?" queried Brenda. "Or is it our perspectives that have helped us appreciate the role of these markers?"

"That's hard to say," said Stan, also feeling the soporific effects of the wine. "I'd say appreciating finitude markers comes first, then my perspective developed from there."

"Me, the opposite," said Brenda. "Perspective first, markers second. I need a way of conceptualizing mortality before I was able to focus on the meaning of finitude markers."

"Me, the opposite, too, I think," added Mandy tentatively. "I needed my perspective on the afterlife before the value of finitude markers became obvious."

Each, in their own way, had found his or her way to the challenge of how to make my-death part of everyday life. Once they had settled on a particular frame, they still needed to find ways of building its presence into their lives. To this end, they had all found the presence of finitude markers central in generating repeated and ongoing connections to my-death.

Meaning and Impacts

As the dinner headed toward its conclusion, all present were aware of one last topic they had neglected to discuss and still needed to cover. How might each of them move forward with their new-found appreciation of my-death, and what would it mean for them in the future?

Brenda carried out the cheesecake she had baked earlier that evening and placed it proudly in the center of the table. Mandy followed her with a bowl of fruit salad and a jug of cream and invited everyone to shovel their choices into their bowls.

Mandy managed a couple of mouthfuls before asking, "So, how are we to understand the different ways we think about death?" She paused to savor another mouthful. "I mean, we can't all be right?"

"I don't think it's about being right or wrong," stated Brenda. "What matters is how you feel about your way of looking at it."

"Hmm," said Leo swallowing a large spoonful of cheesecake. "So, what that implies is that it's a bit like a dinner menu. I like the chicken, Brenda prefers fish, Stan is keen on beef. . . . In the end, what we choose to believe is just a matter of taste?"

"Well, as we've discussed before," replied Brenda, "we might be looking at it in different ways, but the outcome is the same. In the end they each allow us to engage in some form of relationship with death."

"I tell you what," said Stan. "I'd see it more like a toolbox, a conceptual toolbox. Say if I want to remove a troublesome nail, I'd look into my toolkit and find several options for achieving the same thing. I could use a hammer to knock the nail backward and forward until it snaps. I could use my small crowbar to lever it out. If it was a small nail, I could use a set of pliers to pull it out."

Mandy looked up with a quizzical expression. "But that implies that the way I choose to understand my relationship to death is entirely arbitrary; it doesn't really matter which beliefs I buy into. And it suggests I could move easily between these different beliefs: one day looking at it as Brenda does, the next day as Leo does."

"I agree," said Brenda. "It doesn't really resemble a toolkit. It's not something you can flip easily between." She smiled reassuringly across at Stan. "I'd say it's more like a world view; a cluster of interlinked beliefs that fit with your own background, culture, and life circumstances. These are not things you can change easily. The perspective you adopt needs to connect or to resonate with what you already see as familiar."

"I suppose you're right," admitted Stan. "I'm not really likely to be comfortable with the idea of an afterlife because it connects with all the negative things that went on in my early years with religious education. For me it had to be something else."

"Same for me," said Leo, "well, I didn't have much religious education, but life after death seemed an absurd contradiction. I could find no reason to justify thinking that way."

Mandy winced at her son's response. "I know, I know. None of you is with me on this. But it's because of my religious education and because all my life we talked about souls and heaven and God that my recharged belief in an afterlife has become so important."

"I guess that confirms what Brenda is saying," concluded Stan. "I'd say that's a 'yes.' The perspective you end up adopting is not arbitrary. It needs to link with the social and cultural traditions to which you belong."

Their discussion highlighted how relationships involve more than simple connections between two objects. What matters more are the values and meanings that accompany those connections. Each relationship gathers its significance from the broader network of relationships in which it occurs and from the belief structures that underpin that network. When engaging in a relationship with my-death, the meaning of that relationship draws on the broader structures of meaning that imbue it with value and significance. The power of an enabling frame is derived not only from its central idea but also from the extent to which it connects with broader belief systems. As Mandy indicated, her choice of the point-of-transition frame was levered off her wider affiliation to Christian beliefs regarding an afterlife. Her choice was certainly not an arbitrary choice, just as Leo's preference for the essential structures frame was associated with the many exposures and influences that he had encountered. For an enabling frame to do its job, for it to provide a meaningful platform for us to engage with our deaths, it needs to resonate with the complex of cultural and spiritual beliefs which shape how we engage with life.

As a contented fatigue crept across the four diners, they had just enough time to consider one further aspect of the meaning of engagement with my-death: namely, whether it had improved their lives in any way.

Mandy pushed her empty dessert bowl forward, leaned back in her chair, and allowed a contented look to spread across her face. She sighed. "Well, I'd just like to point out, up to a year ago, we were all finding it hard to think or talk about death."

"Yes, that's right," said Brenda. "Each of us has, in our own way, found a path through this to form a new and closer relationship."

"Okay," said Mandy taking another sip of wine. "So what have we gained for our trouble? I mean, are our lives any better from getting closer to death?"

"Hmm, that's a thought-provoking question," said Stan. "Are we any better off?"

"I'll tell you what I've gained," continued Mandy. "I'm no longer scared of death. Before I was terrified to even think about it. I'd even close others down in case it infected me." She nodded toward Leo. "But now I feel less scared, more relaxed, more at peace with the world."

"Hmm," said Leo pensively. "For me it has been like an awakening, like coming out of a dark tunnel into the light. I'm different from the rest of you; you've all had more time to think about these things. The real meaning of death didn't hit me until Aunty Sue's funeral. But, from there, I reckon I've moved very fast."

"That's an understatement," said Stan. "You've managed to cover more territory in several months than I was able to do over seventy years. Perhaps I'm a bit slow, but since my heart attack, my appreciation of life all around me has intensified; everything seems more vibrant, more imbued with meaning. Also, with death by my side, I feel I have a better handle on what's important to me. Of course, I can say that because I'm so much older than the rest of you. But really, I could have started this a lot earlier."

"That just leaves me," said Brenda. "What have I gained?" She was tapping the stem of her wineglass. "What I've gained is something I never expected. I thought since I worked with death I knew as much as I needed. But I hadn't really faced my own death. Now, prodded by you, I've explored what this means; I feel I have my own relationship with it, and this has given me a new basis for talking to patients about their relationships with death."

Stan could feel a drowsiness spreading through his body. He glanced at his watch. "Ooh, it's after ten, I'll really need to go; Winston will be worrying about me." He stood up, stretched, and yawned. "Look, I've had such a good time this evening. I'm so grateful for the work you've all done and for acknowledging my recovery. Thank you all, so much. But now my body tells me I must retire." He walked awkwardly toward the back door, glancing back to see three smiles beaming back their farewells.

In retrospect, their refreshed relationships to my-death were seen as positive and productive. They also recognized that this positive value was not apparent before finding the frame that suited them. The next chapter will focus in more detail on the benefits of a relationship to my-death and how this might be promoted with people generally.

Notes

1. J. Sexton, "The semantics of death and dying: Metaphor and mortality," *ETC: A Review of General Semantics* (54:3, 333–45, 1997).
2. B. Spall, S. Read, and D, Chantry, "Metaphor: Exploring its origins and therapeutic use in death, dying and bereavement," *International Journal of Palliative Nursing* (7:7, 345–53, 2001).
3. L. Ross and H. Pollio, "Metaphors of death," *Omega: Journal of Death and Dying* (23:4, 291–307, 1991).
4. Stan started with Heidegger's ideas but developed them into a more personal and experiential perspective.
5. While Mandy missed picking up on it, Stan was signaling an important link between the nature of death and the nature of suffering. Suffering is both something we all encounter in the course of life and something we anticipate at the end of life. Stan was positioning suffering as a further space in which we encounter finitude. For a review of the links between dying and suffering, see A. Kellehear, "On dying and human suffering," *Palliative Medicine* (23:5, 388–397, 2009).

11

What's to Gain?

During their meal to celebrate Stan's recovery, the four companions all agreed that their engagement with my-death was a good thing. Indeed, the six previous chapters have taken this for granted with repeated reference to life-enhancing benefits. But is this the case? Does engaging with my-death lead to improvements in the quality and meaningfulness of our lives? Some writers definitely do see it as having strong psychological, emotional, and spiritual benefits. For example, as the Austrian psychiatrist and Holocaust survivor Viktor Frankl (1952) pointed out,

> How often we hear the argument that death does away with the meaning of life altogether. That in the end all man's works are meaningless, since death ultimately destroys them. Now, does death really decrease the mean- ingfulness of life? On the contrary. For what would our lives be like if they were not finite in time, but infinite? If we were immortal, we could le- gitimately postpone every action forever. It would be of no consequence whether or not we did a thing now . . . But in the face of death as absolute finis to our future and boundary to our possibilities, we are under the im- perative of utilizing our lifetimes to the utmost—not letting the singular opportunities whose "finite" sum constitutes the whole of life—pass by unused.[1]

Frankl was strongly of the view that a relationship with my-death is life- enhancing because, without the finality of death, the meaningfulness of everyday experience would be absorbed into an amorphous and featureless desert.

By way of contrast, others have argued that pursuing a relationship to my-death could entail a range of negative and demoralizing consequences, particularly with regard to its potential impacts on mental well-being. For example, the renowned Danish philosopher Søren Kierkegaard (2004, 1849) described some of the ambiguously negative consequences of engaging with my-death as follows:

. . . eternity asks you . . . just one thing: whether you have lived in despair or not, whether so in despair that you did not know that you were in despair, or in such a way that you bore this sickness concealed deep inside you as your gnawing secret, under your heart like the fruit of a sinful love, or in such a way that, a terror to others, you raged in despair. If then, if you have lived in despair, then whatever else you won or lost, for you everything is lost, eternity does not acknowledge you, it never knew you, or, still more dreadful, it knows you as you are known, it manacles you to yourself in despair![2]

While Kierkegaard's philosophy was anything but avoidant of the topic of my-death, what he says here captures some of the sense of why engaging with my-death could be deemed pointless and unnecessarily distressing. We have already encountered this negativity in many places: its impenetrable nothingness, the scariness of not knowing when and how my-dying will occur, and the threat it poses to all that exists, including lovedones. As Mandy claimed in earlier chapters, the negativity of my-death has the potential to pollute the mind with morbid thoughts which could easily build into a general negative outlook on life resulting in longer term mental states such as anxiety or depression.

This chapter turns its back on such negativity and explores the potential of my-death connectivity first, in improving our quality of life; second, in heightening our commitment to fundamental values; and, third, in helping with our passage through the end of life.

Quality of Life

Let's turn first to the positive life-enhancing aspects of pursuing an ongoing relationship with my-death. The various branches of the "psy" sciences—most notably psychology, psychotherapy, and psychiatry—have grappled with the role of my-death as an enhancer of well-being and self-actualization. For example, Giampaolo Moraglia (2004) examined how prominent psychologists—such as William James, B. F. Skinner, and Stanley Hall—approached the subject of death in their writings. He argued that their views converged in a number of ways, but, most importantly,

the overwhelming majority of these writers support the view that a confrontation with one's mortality is not morbid and inimical to life; on the contrary, it may constitute one of the necessary preconditions for psychological growth. Moreover, the appreciation of one's finiteness, far from casting a pall upon the meaningfulness of one's life, is a necessary constituent of it.[3]

In the same vein, two psychotherapists, Robert Firestone and Joyce Catlett (2009), explored how improved death awareness and reduced defensiveness can open up opportunities for improving one's quality of life.

The less defended individual feels more alive, has the opportunity to experience more freedom and independence, and has a greater chance to evolve and fulfill his or her human potential. Making this choice is what the authors refer to as life-affirming death awareness.[4]

Despite the confidence of these assertions, surprisingly little research is available to support the idea of my-death awareness as life-enhancing. A few studies have approached it indirectly by talking with people who are working with the dying. For example, Shane Sinclair (2011) interviewed six leaders and twenty-four clinicians involved in end-of-life care in Canada and found that, among other themes, they had all experienced significant encounters with other-death early in their lives and claimed that working with the dying had positively transformed the way they lived their lives by

teaching them to live in the present, cultivate spiritual life and reflect deeply on the continuity of life. . . .
    Mortality was not seen by participants simply as an event at the end of life but, rather, as an ever present, moment-by-moment reality embedded across the continuity of life.[5]

However, it is worth noting that end-of-life care professionals might be viewed as a group who already see death awareness as fascinating and see themselves as having acquired a developed understanding of death issues, and, accordingly, this does not shed much light on how ordinary members of society might perceive it.

Brenda dropped in on Stan, curious to see how he had found the dinner two nights before. She found him in his backyard attending to his potted plants with Winston sniffing with interest the soil he was prodding.

"Stan, you're taking it easy, aren't you?" she queried. "We can't have you keeling over again."

"No heavy lifting with these small things," stated Stan as he beckoned her over to sit down at his cast-iron garden seat. Winston curled up next to them. "That was quite an evening you all put on. I found it very moving. I didn't know what to say...."

"Well, after all you've done for us, we had to acknowledge your recovery."

"You know what, Brenda?" said Stan wiping sweat from his face with a small towel, "Ever since my heart attack, I sense death all around; everything speaks to me of my mortality: I see it in nature, in other people and in my own body. But, strangely, rather than making me more nervous, I now feel less worried about it because I feel my death is . . . well, it's like a friend; a helpful friend whose encouraging me to enjoy life more."

"Yeah, I must admit, since clarifying how I think about death I'm not only feeling more relaxed about it but calmer about life as a whole."

"When I left the hospital and got through the worst phases of my recovery, my outlook changed; I became less worried about the distant future and more interested in the little things."

"Funny how a scare like that can shock you into sanity."

"I now feel every moment's a gift. I'm enjoying the most mundane things: the sun's warmth, the blossoming of flowers in my garden, Winston's little nudges. . . . It's almost as though the little things are shining more radiantly than the big things."

"Hmm, more at peace with the world," concluded Brenda leaning over to pat Winston.

"Don't get me wrong, I'm still scared of what I might go through when I finally get around to dying, but, strangely enough, I'm not scared of death itself. Everything now seems like a bonus; a bonus I don't really deserve. When it comes time for me to die, I expect my awareness of it to be just an extension of what I'm thinking now."

Stan and Brenda's unfalteringly positive view of engaging with my-death is not shared by everyone. One line of research has uncovered a very different story. Indeed, the most consistent and significant effort to research the psychological impacts of such awareness has emerged under the banner of "terror management theory" and incorporates more than thirty years of research involving hundreds of university studies—mainly in psychology departments—and occurring in many different locations around the world.[6]

Terror management theory views thoughts of my-death as playing a vital role in many of the diverse aspects of our mental world including self-esteem, prejudice, aggression, and nationalism.[7] At its heart it argues that awareness of the inevitability and finality of my-death generates unwanted existential terror which we then strive to control by means of beliefs which are set into internalized cultural worldviews which then help us to buffer and protect ourselves from this overwhelming anxiety. These worldviews typically incorporate beliefs about us continuing to exist, in some form, beyond our death. Alongside these beliefs we derive self-esteem from our efforts to live up to the values and standards prescribed by these worldviews. These two ingredients, worldviews and self-esteem, operate in tandem. Together they help us manage those overwhelming feelings of helplessness and terror associated with thinking about my-death, and we achieve this by means of an elaborate system of psychological mechanisms that protect us from thinking about it.

Terror management theorists have looked closely at the ways we suppress thoughts about my-death and have identified a wide range of what they call "symbolic defenses." Tom Pyszczynski and colleagues (1999) have divided these defenses into two clusters, proximal and distal.[8] *Proximal mechanisms* involve conscious, rational, and immediate attempts to push contemplation of my-death into the future by favoring thoughts that deny the inevitability of death. Examples of such thoughts include ideas of an afterlife or viewing life as continuing on forever. *Distal mechanisms* involve more indirect symbolic processes by modifying how we see ourselves in terms of worldviews and self-esteem. They occur at a more abstract level and involve evaluating one's life with regard to more culturally valued attributes—such as intelligence and creativity—and fulfillment of key social roles—such as being a doctor or a parent. As the initial line of defense, proximal mechanisms tend to occur at a similar level to where we might be feeling threatened, as when, for example, a smoker denies the risk factors associated with tobacco-related lung disease. Distal mechanisms attempt to diffuse a threat at a more abstract and long-term level by, for example, progressively building up self-esteem according to key culturally derived values, such as fairness and kindness, and thereby making life seem more purposeful and meaningful.[9]

A second key concept in terror management theory is "mortality salience," and it refers to the extent to which we are responsive to the many subtle cues and reminders of my-death which constantly infuse our lives. These cues approximate to what in earlier chapters I have referred to as *finitude markers*.

They involve sudden, unexpected thoughts about mortality in response to cues such as the death of loved ones, life-threatening incidents, or just images reminding us of our transience. These cues matter because they have the potential to threaten our cultural worldviews and self-esteem and thereby reduce our capacity to protect ourselves from paralyzing death anxiety.[10]

Experiments in this area typically involve participants being asked to complete packets of what are described to them as personality questionnaires. Embedded in these packets are invitations to briefly write something about either my-death or a non–death-related topic—the latter intended as a comparison or control group. The contrast between those who are primed with thoughts about my-death and those who are not primed provides researchers with the means to compare the extent to which priming people to their own mortality increases the strength of their cultural worldviews and self-esteem.[11] For example, Mark Landau and colleagues (2011) conducted three experiments in this style with undergraduate students where mortality salience was manipulated, first, by embedding death-related words into a letter grid puzzle (e.g., "burial" or "corpse"); second, by asking additional questions about death following a life goal-setting task; and, third, by asking how life could have been different if an influential event had not occurred. In all three experiments, mortality salience participants scored significantly higher than controls in terms of motivation to imbue their everyday actions with meaning, thus supporting the main tenets of terror management theory.[12] Studies of this type have been numerous. Brian Burke and colleagues (2010) conducted a meta-analysis combining data from 277 experiments measuring mortality salience and concluded that the mortality salience hypothesis

> is robust and produces moderate to large effects across a wide variety of MS [mortality salience] manipulations as well as attitudinal, behavioral, and cognitive DVs [dependent variables].[13]

Terror management theory has found applications in a wide range of areas, too wide to cover in this book. However, to give a taste of these applications, Bassett and Connolly (2011) explored the effects of mortality salience on racial bias by using the standard design discussed earlier then asking their psychology students to read two identical stories about immigrants who entered the United States without proper legal documents, except that one was about Ben Johnson from Vancouver and the other about Carlos Suarez from Mexico City. They were then asked about the extent to which they thought such immigrants undermine US cultural and economic systems. They found that reminders of my-death tended to intensify reactions to culturally dissimilar targets such as white Americans responding more negatively to the Latino story.[14] Similar studies on racism, intergroup tension, and global conflict have yielded similar results.[15] What these studies are suggesting is that by increasing our confidence in our particular worldviews, we manage to hold our death anxiety at bay. But when living alongside people who favor different worldviews, we are likely to feel unsettled because their different beliefs challenge the absolute validity of one's worldview and thereby undermine the effectiveness of the strategy we are using to buffer our death anxiety.

Brenda carried two glasses of water across to Stan's garden table. She sat down and commented, "I can see how a close encounter with death helps put life into perspective, but it's not like that for everybody."

Stan nodded. "No, I can remember a time when talking about my death was the last thing I wanted to do. I don't think it was a conscious reaction; just that whenever the topic or thoughts about the topic cropped up, I felt uneasy . . . uneasy the way you feel when you avoid talking to someone close about something very sensitive, such as a betrayal or a mental health issue."

"Like the proverbial elephant in the room?"

"Yes, but lacking any specific focus," said Stan smiling. "I guess it's more like the elephant becomes the room."

"So, what if I was to keep harping on about death?" asked Brenda. "What if I had kept pushing through all your diversion tactics? How would you have reacted then?"

"I'd have become very annoyed; not only because I was uneasy but because you'd made it obvious both to me and others that I was avoiding the topic."

"It wouldn't have done any harm."

"I dunno about that. Thinking back to how I was at the time, being forced to talk about death could have upset a very fine balance. At different times in my life I've been prone to depression, particularly after my time in Vietnam. Forced conversations might have triggered some unwanted thoughts and pushed me back into a depressive state. I'm not sure you can assume it's automatically a good thing."

"But for us four," said Brenda, "none of us was pushed into thinking about death?"

"No, but entry into these conversations hasn't been easy. Both you and Mandy had to endure considerable emotional turmoil in finding your way, and I nearly died as part of the process."

"Hmm, but it has been worth it. I think we all agree that our different ways of connecting with death have led us to appreciate life differently."

As implied by the term "terror management," my-death awareness is generally seen as contributing to negative and destructive psychological processes. Indeed, in a review of such impacts, Jacob Juhl and Clay Routledge (2016) identified studies that demonstrated how my-death awareness could result in increased anxiety and lower self-confidence, particularly for those who have a lower sense of self-worth and who lack other psychological buffers.[16] But their conclusion is controversial. Mario Mikulincer and colleagues (2003) had already opened these processes up by pointing out the important role close relationships play in reducing my-death anxiety. In interpreting their findings they claimed that

> close relationships not only protect individuals from concrete and actual threats and dangers but also provide a symbolic shield against the awareness of one's finitude. In addition the findings . . . emphasize the dynamic interplay between close relationships, cultural worldview validation, and self-esteem [. . . and] emphasize a psychological equation between threats to relationship maintenance and death concerns.[17]

Following this lead, Kenneth Vail and colleagues (2012) looked more closely at the potential of my-death awareness to contribute to both personally and socially beneficial outcomes. In their review of the evidence, they distinguished between the conscious and nonconscious effects of thinking about my-death. At a conscious level, thoughts about my-death can motivate us to enhance our physical health and reprioritize important life-goals. At a nonconscious level, such awareness can move us to live up to our primary values—such as justice and compassion—and build positive close relationships.[18]

Philip Cozzolino (2006) has approached the negativity of terror management theory from another angle. He drew a distinction between the narrow psychological focus on mortality salience pursued by most studies and what he refers to as "death reflection." Looking at people who survive serious trauma or who have had near-death experiences, he pointed to another line of literature that highlights how people benefit psychologically following their trauma. He argued that posttraumatic growth occurs where

> contemplating the immediacy of one's death, rather than engaging mortality only in the abstract, can systematically guide one from relative existential darkness to a place of self-awareness and growth.[19]

In a later study, Cozzolino and colleagues (2014) asked 185 Californians to fill in questionnaires on fear of death and a range of measures of self-realization and well-being. They found that people with lower levels of fear and avoidance of death were more likely to have an enhanced sense of self and stronger existential well-being. They concluded that stronger engagement with death leads to a stronger, healthier "actual-self," by which they meant a self that is "personally valued, clearly conceived, efficacious, and that has intrinsic meaning and purpose."[20]

It is hard not to be impressed by the sheer volume of effort that has gone into researching terror management theory.[21] The plentiful and wide-ranging studies have demonstrated the powerful role my-death awareness is likely to be playing in many aspects of our psychological make-up, including personal motivation, self-concepts, and social beliefs. As acknowledged by the researchers themselves, their methods are constrained by many of the same limitations that afflict experimental research in psychology generally, such as a heavy reliance on student participants, the problematic validity of attitudinal questionnaires, and the arbitrary ways we might respond to abstract and hypothetical scenarios. Initially the research focused on the negativity of the "terror" component of the theory. However, as the research has advanced, a more positive and life-enhancing picture is emerging, particularly when they include more of the existential and social dimensions of my-death awareness.

Life Revaluation

Another assertion regarding the merits of pursuing a relationship with my-death, and one hinted at in the previous section, concerns its capacity to act as a catalyst for evaluating or revaluing one's outlook on life. The Finnish philosopher Sara Heinämaa (2015) has made use of Husserl's phenomenology to explore the creative or generative potential offered by such a relationship.

[In] so far as death is not an event for us, we should not relate to it as we relate to threatening worldly happenings, that is, by precautions, preparations, provisions, supplies, insurances and guidelines. . . . Rather than trying to bar against a gigantic misfortune and a final catastrophe or to minimize the effects of such imaginary events we should aim at controlling the focus of our attention here and now. . . .

. . . the threatening character of death depends on its sense as an interruption. Clarity is gained by noticing that the dimensions of our lives that are most severely threatened by interruptions are its progressive dimensions, that is, our practical and goal-positing activities.[22]

When thoughts of my-death intrude, they throw into question plans and expectations for the future, but, in the process, this also opens up opportunities for reappraising life goals.

After Brenda had departed, Stan resumed his potting, only to be interrupted by Mandy, also curious about how he'd found the dinner.

"Ah, Mandy, come and sit down." Stan led her over to the garden seat. "Brenda was just here discussing what we gain from thinking about death."

"That's a good topic, particularly at the moment."

"Ah, yes, if it's the dinner you're referring to, I must say it was a marvelous event. Thank you so much for putting it on."

"Actually, it wasn't the dinner but what happened afterward that mattered more to me."

Stan raised his eyebrows and smiled. "Go on."

"Well, the Sunday morning after the dinner, I felt all wrung out and wanted to get away from the people and the house and everything. I drove out into the countryside to a river walkway that I knew would be mostly deserted, then I just wandered off along the path."

"It's nice to get away like that from time to time."

"During the first hour my head was churning with everything we'd been discussing the night before; all our various ideas, positions. and arguments. After a while these merged together into an amorphous mass, then, in my mind's eye, I conjured up the presence of my death; I put it there, a few yards in front of me, standing there staring at me."

"I'm not going to ask you what death looked like. I'm assuming you're meaning an imaginative, symbolic figure?"

"Yeah, I suppose so. But I did imagine it saying something to me." Mandy glanced nervously across at Stan. "It was calling on me to think about where I stood; what matters most to me and what I want out of my future."

"So, I guess that wasn't too hard given all our recent talk about death?"

"I said to death that what matters most are my relationships with my family, my friends, my work colleagues, and, of course, you, Leo, and Brenda. Death didn't respond. So I thought about it again. I said my mental and physical well-being mattered, as does being happy and content with what I do during the day. Death remained expressionless. I was wondering what it was after. So I spontaneously said I wanted to be as much as possible in touch with, no, passionately in touch with life and all that comes with it. At this Death smiled." Mandy paused and stared at Stan with her mouth open. "And then I felt this amazing sense of correctness sweep over me."

Mandy's shift to fully embracing the afterlife and her more relaxed stance on death had prompted her to review not only the meaning of my-death in her life but also its relationship to other things she held dear.

Other researchers have used analysis of in-depth interviews as a window onto what my-death might mean in our lives. For example, Agnieszka Widera-Wysoczańska (1999) interviewed twelve Polish women about how they experienced their relationships to their own deaths. Among other issues, including the negative impacts of death, her informants described how images of death motivated them to improve their lives.

> They did this by focusing on their faith in themselves and recognizing internal opportunities available and that it was important to enjoy their lives, create some distance from negative events and influences, focus on living more fully in the moment, more intensively, and give more serious attention to their psychological state or mental health.[23]

Interestingly, and in line with the orientation of this book, half of those Widera-Wysoczańska interviewed described my-death as a "life companion."[24]

Some researchers have approached the disruptive potential of my-death from another angle by exploring the processes people use to make meaning of their own life following the death of loved ones. James Gillies (2006) reviewed the typical meaning-making activities following a bereavement and pointed out how losses which are difficult to understand and accept, losses which seem inconsistent with understandings before the loss, can be highly disruptive and are likely to prompt a search for meaning.[25] With a more specific focus, Janoff-Bulman and McPherson (1997) explored the literature on how meanings are impacted by sudden and traumatic bereavements. They theorized that the bereaved

> *experience the pain of shattered assumptions and increased awareness of their own vulnerability; they know human outcomes can be random and meaningless. Yet they also experience the pleasure of a newfound appreciation of life and sense of value and meaning in their daily existence. . . . Against the backdrop of a meaningless world, survivors create a life of meaning.[26]*

The importance of meaning-making was explored further by Güler Boyraz and colleagues (2015) who identified ways in which bereavement is influenced by what they called "neutral acceptance" or seeing death as a natural and inevitable part of life. They surveyed 160 people recently bereaved regarding grief, death attitudes, and meaning in life. They found that those who saw death as a natural part of life had a stronger sense of meaning in their lives and that this appeared to help in lessening the negative effects of their bereavement.

However, while some researchers have explored the contribution of my-death awareness to the processes of bereavement and end of life, the way this works in the course of a whole lifetime has yet to be clarified. It seems plausible that closer contact with my-death during different periods of one's life would prompt a re-valuation of life-goals and a reassessment what is seen as important and meaningful. As suggested earlier, such moments can interrupt the normal taken-for-granted flow of what is going on and, in the process, generate moments of questioning that challenge current attachments.

Preparation for End-of-Life

Who knows how each of us will handle that period toward the end of our lives? For some of us it will come quickly and unexpectedly, leaving little room for engaging with the prospect of dying. For people like Stan, the threat of death comes and goes. For others of us, where the news of a terminal condition comes well in advance of our final exit, we will have a great deal of time to think about what it means.

But will we?

During end-of-life period, many things require attention before that final moment. Loved ones will be reacting to their sadness and anticipated grief; they will need support and reassurance. Management of the illness will occupy energy and time, including the many medical consultations, endless adjustments in medication, and challenges in adapting to the paraphernalia of palliative care. Then come fears of how death will occur: fears of unbearable pain, fears of seeing the grief in the eyes of family, fears of disablement, of depending on others, of deteriorating mobility, and of impaired mental capacity, and, of course, overriding fears of loss of dignity.

On top of this are the subtle and not-so-subtle shifts in social identity. Friends and acquaintances look at you and respond to you differently. They see you as occupying a different category of person: someone dealing with unnatural forces, someone in distress, and someone without a future. They have difficulties knowing what to say, and many choose to keep their distance. And bit-by-bit the way others see you seeps into your mind and infects how you see yourself: you begin to think of yourself as different from normal people. You are also faced with determining arrangements for after you die: The funeral, how will that be conducted? Financial affairs, how will your inheritance be distributed? Your legacy, how will you be remembered by your children, by your community, even by the public? So much will be demanding your attention; so much that has the potential to compete and, perhaps, eclipse how you are engaging with and responding to my-death.

With other tasks at end-of-life likely to crowd out engagement with my-death, people entering that phase are likely to be better equipped for what they encounter should they bring with them an already assembled relationship with my-death. Prior involvement with any of the four enabling frames, or other permutations, would provide the basis for a stronger engagement with my-death at end-of-life.

Leo found Brenda curled up on the couch in the living room reading a book. He settled into the armchair and declared unceremoniously. "Yesterday I was thinking of what it would be like to die in a head-on collision." He looked across at Brenda with a faint smile. "In that split second before the crash, I'd see the other car flying toward me and I would know what's coming. At that moment I would be poised right in front of my own death. What would I be thinking? How would I welcome the inevitable?"

Brenda looked up from her book, surprised by Leo's unsolicited tirade. "Hmm, I would hate to go that way," she said, grimacing as she put her book down and sat up. "It would be a missed opportunity. Even if I had already established a strong relationship with death, a sudden exit would deny me time to process what's going on."

"But does that really matter? What difference does it make how you face it in the end?"

"Okay, get this," said Brenda, pausing to collect her thoughts. "I was talking this over with Stan a few days ago, and he actually declared to me he was pleased he'd had his heart attack; not pleased with all the pain and discomfort, but pleased for what it prompted in him afterward. See, he feels lucky because it gave him a chance to rethink his relationship to death, and now he says he's in a much better space and more prepared to face it when it finally comes."

"It might be quite different when he actually does face it," observed Leo. "But, I take your point. I can see how this worked for Mom." He raised his legs and wrapped his arms around his knees. "A few months ago, before Mom changed, she refused to talk about death, and, for whatever reason, she forbade me from even thinking about it. Now look at her. She can't get enough."

"Yes, it's quite a change, and she's really pleased with her shift in perspective."

"So let's suppose Mom was told she had cancer and only had three months to live. Let's suppose this happened before her change. I reckon she'd probably spend the first two months trying not to think about it, and only slowly come round to talking about it in the last month . . . and then it would be too late for her to make much headway."

"Actually, I do see that sometimes at work. I see patients who are not ready to talk about their death until just before they die, and then they have no time to work it out. It strikes me that it's far better to sort out your relationship to death well before you get told you're going to die because, that way, you already have a platform from which to engage."

The question of whether a more developed understanding of my-death leads to a better quality of dying has not attracted much research interest. Some researchers have looked at whether improved understanding during the end of life makes any difference. For example, Barney Glaser and Anselm Strauss (1966), in their book *Awareness of Dying*, reported on observations and interviews with people in hospitals who were dying and the relationships they were having with those around them, including family members and care professionals.[27] They named the places where these interactions were taking place as "awareness contexts," which they then divided further into "closed awareness," where patients were unaware of their status; "suspected awareness," where the topic of death was implicit; "mutual pretense awareness," where all involved pretended death was not occurring; and "open awareness," where all parties acknowledged the patient's condition as terminal. For each awareness context they described in detail the social interactions that were occurring and what they meant for the people involved. For instance, they explored the expectations of nurses and doctors that patients die in "acceptable" ways and occasions when patients are admonished for not displaying appropriate levels of dignity and grace. They also highlighted the strengths of open awareness contexts in allowing all concerned to prepare and adapt to the approaching end, but, at the same time, they acknowledged how openness could be undesirably distressing for some, particularly those with strong fears of death.[28]

Other researchers have looked at the spiritual and existential processes at end of life. Christine Melin-Johansson and colleagues (2012) reviewed seventeen studies looking into the existential concerns of those with life-threatening illnesses and the people who cared for them, all of whom identified the need for both patients and their families to have support in navigating their existential issues. Eunmi Ahn and colleagues (2013) asked 345 Korean patients being admitted to palliative care units to complete a range of questionnaires on their views regarding quality of death and illness awareness.[29] They found that more than two-thirds of their sample were aware that their illness was terminal, and, compared to those unaware of their status, they were more likely to experience a better quality of death involving a stronger sense of hope and autonomy. On this basis they recommended "careful disclosure of the terminal status," particularly for those from Asian cultural backgrounds.

Despite suggestions from end-of-life research that an open relationship with my-death contributes to a better quality of dying, the focus of this book extends wider than dying to include death as an aspect of one's entire lifetime. The accent is on looking for ways to engage with my-death long before the end of life.

Brenda glanced across at Leo, who was now slumped back in the armchair.

"At your age, dying must seem a long way off?"

"No, no, as you may have noticed, I've been trying to get closer to death; to reach out and touch it and entice it into being part of my life." Leo pointed nonchalantly in Brenda's direction. "But what about *you*? You're constantly in touch with it because you work with it. Doesn't it feel close to *you*?"

Brenda smiled at his cheeky emphasis. "Maybe, but lately I've been shocked by my lack of understanding and by how quickly that can change. A few months ago I thought I had it all worked out. I knew exactly how I'd handle my final months: plenty of people, plenty of talk about death, and lots of reflection on what my life had meant. But then all our conversations made me aware that I wasn't really clear about how I thought of my own death and that I hadn't managed to draw it close."

"Well, has that changed?"

"I guess, on the surface, I'd handle it much the same, but deeper down I think I'd experience things quite differently. See, what's different is I now have a well-assembled relationship with my death which guides me in listening to others talking about their deaths."

"So you'd like them to see death the way you do?" said Leo with a mischievous grin.

"No, on the contrary, it provides what seems to me a secure platform for appreciating what other people are saying and responding in a way that respects their views."

"I can see that. Same for me. Having my own way of looking at death makes me less defensive and more ready to accept other's views."

"Yes, when I finally said goodbye to notions of a beyond death and moved to embracing death as something I do or perform in the course of living, when I saw things this way, I felt more grounded in the way I see things. But I still knew this was a way of seeing things and that other ways of seeing were just as possible and just as valid. I was just more confident in myself and, at the same time, more willing to hear about other perspectives."

"Hmm, but this could all change when the doctor says you only have two months to live."

"Yes, maybe, but I'd like to think that my journey of connecting with death is ongoing and shaped by many things. I also assume that knowing when I'm going to die will intensify this relationship, but not change the framework I've developed for understanding it."

While we lack strong evidence that adopting any of the discussed enabling frames leads to improvements in both living and dying, I am, clearly, from the momentum of this book, of the view that engaging in a prior relationship with my-death would be of benefit at the end of life. Some advantages immediately spring to mind. If I manage to establish a firm relationship with my-death via one of the enabling frames, I am less likely to need to work through habitual patterns of avoidance and denial which are likely to complicate and delay all those aspects of death I will be needing to face. It would be terrible to spend the first three months avoiding any discussion of death leaving only two weeks for open discussion; I would be poorly prepared for my final moments. Another advantage follows logically from much of what has been presented so far. An established relationship to my-death would reduce or perhaps eliminate the need to deal with this area, leaving me free to focus on the other complex challenges associated with the process of dying. If I do need to think about it, prior experience would make it familiar territory; it would simply be an extension of what I had been doing for many years. I would not be starting from scratch; I would enter equipped with preformed abilities in thinking and talking about my-death, and this would help me in responding and adapting to what I encounter.

Notes

1. Viktor Frankl, *The Doctor and the Soul: From Psychotherapy to Logotherapy* (New York: Alfred A. Knopf, 1952) pp. 72–73 (author's original emphasis removed).
2. S. Kierkegaard, *The Sickness Unto Death* (Penguin Classics, 2004, 1849).
3. G. Moraglia, "On facing death: Views of some prominent psychologists," *Journal of Humanistic Psychology* (44:3, 337–57, 2004) p. 355.
4. R. Firestone and J. Catlett, *Beyond Death Anxiety* (New York: Springer, 2009) p. 6 (authors' original emphasis removed).
5. S. Sinclair, "Impact of death and dying on the personal lives and practices of palliative and hospice care professionals," *Canadian Medical Association Journal* (183:2, 180–87, 2011) pp. 182–83.
6. A summary of more than 300 studies up to 2005 is provided by T. Pyszczynski et al., "On the unique psychological import of the human awareness of mortality," *Psychological Inquiry* (17:4, 328–56, 2006).
7. For example, on its relevance to mental well-being, see A. Lewis, "Terror management theory applied clinically," *Death Studies* (38:6, 412–17, 2014).
8. T. Pyszczynski, J. Greenberg, and S. Solomon, "A dual-process model of defense against conscious and unconscious death-related thoughts," *Psychological Review* (106:4, 835–45, 1999).

9. More detail on defenses can be found in L. Harvell and G. Nisbett, eds., *Denying Death: An Interdisciplinary Approach to Terror Management Theory* (New York: Routledge, 2016) and in J. Arndt and M. Vess, "Tales from existential oceans," *Social and Personality Psychology Compass* (2:2, 909–28, 2008).

10. More detail on mortality salience is discussed by R. Neimeyer, J. Wittkowski, and R. Moser in "Psychological research on death attitudes," *Death Studies* (28:4 309–40, 2004), and by V. Florian, M. Mikulincer, and G. Hirschberger in "An existentialist view on mortality salience effects," *British Journal of Social Psychology* (40:3, 437–53, 2001).

11. Experiments on terror management theory are summarized by M. Mikulincer and V. Florian in "The complex mulifaceted nature of the fear of personal death," in A. Tomer et al., eds., *Existential and Spiritual Issues in Death Attitudes* (New York: Laurence Erlbaum, 2013), pp. 29–64.

12. M. Landau, S. Kosloff, and B. Schmeichel, "Imbuing everyday actions with meaning in response to existential threat," *Self and Identity* (10:1, 64–76, 2011).

13. B. Burke, A. Martens, and E. Faucher, "Two decades of terror management theory," *Personality and Social Psychology Review* (14:2, 155–95, 2010) p. 187.

14. J. Bassett and J. Connelly, "Terror management and reactions to undocumented immigrants," *Journal of Social Psychology* (151:2, 117–20, 2011).

15. For example, see E. Jonas and I. Fritsche, "Destined to die but not to wage war," *American Psychologist* (68:7, 543–48, 2013), and A. Abdollahi, C. Henthorn, and T. Pyszczynski, "Experimental peace psychology," *Behavioral Sciences of Terrorism & Political Aggression* (2, 30–37, 2010).

16. J. Juhl and C. Routledge, "Putting the terror in terror management theory," *Current Directions in Psychological Science* (25:2, 99–103, 2016).

17. M. Mikulincer, V. Florian, and G. Hirschberger, "The existential function of close relationships," *Personality and Social Psychology Review* (7:1, 20–40, 2003) p. 37.

18. K. Vail et al., "When death is good for life."

19. P. Cozzolino, "Death contemplation, growth, and defense," *Psychological Inquiry* (17:4, 278–87, 2006) p. 284.

20. P. Cozzolino, L. Blackie, and L. Meyers, "Self-related consequences of death fear and death denial," *Death Studies* (38:6, 418–22, 2014) p. 421.

21. Terror management theory was preceded by and links to the earlier psychological research on fear of death covered in Chapter 4.

22. Sara Heinämaa, "The many senses of death," in O. Hakola et al., eds., *Death and Mortality: For Individual to Communal Perspectives* (Helsinki Collegium for Advanced Studies, 2015) pp. 100–18, at 110–11.

23. A. Widera-Wysoczańska, "Everyday awareness of death," *Journal of Humanistic Psychology* (39:3, 73–92, 1999) p. 88.

24. Ibid., p. 84.

25. J. Gillies and R. Neimeyer, "Loss, grief, and the search for significance," *Journal of Constructivist Psychology* (19:1, 31–65, 2006), particularly see p. 54.

26. R. Janoff-Bulman and C. Frantz, "The impact of trauma on meaning," in M. Power and C. Brewin, eds., *The Transformation of Meaning in Psychological Therapies Practice* (Hoboken: Wiley, 1997) pp. 99–106, at p. 103.

27. B. Glaser and A. Strauss, *Awareness of Dying* (New Brunswick: Aldine Transaction, 1966). They are renowned as the fathers of grounded theory research, now a widely used form of qualitative method often also employed in researching death and dying.

28. The issue over whether open discussion of dying is suitable for all patients or whether conditional and graduated forms of openness are better is covered by D. Field and G. Copp in "Communication and awareness about dying in the 1990s," *Palliative Medicine* (13:6, 459–68, 1999).

29. E. Ahn et al., "The impact of awareness of terminal illness on quality of death and care decision making," *Psycho-Oncology* (22:12, 2771–78, 2013).

12

Applications

The ancient Greek philosopher Epicurus famously claimed that "death is nothing to us" thereby implying that needless my-death anxiety and pointless conversations and ruminations about it add little to what we aim to get out of life.

> *Become accustomed to the belief that death is nothing to us. For all good and evil consists in sensation, but death is deprivation of sensation . . . So death, the most terrifying of ills, is nothing to us, since so long as we exist death is not with us; but when death comes, then we do not exist. It does not then concern either the living or the dead, since for the former it is not, and the latter are no more.[1]*

In this book I am clearly disagreeing with Epicurus's pragmatic position. I have argued that an ongoing relationship to my-death is a possibility—admittedly an indirect and figurative possibility—but still a possibility, and that, in the long run, pursuing such a relationship can be beneficial.

Besides, whichever way it is approached, inside the arena of conversations about death lurks the unspeakable presence of my-death. Contact with it is unavoidable. Any discussion on the nature of life and death will inevitably traverse its presence and, perhaps, touch briefly on its relevance. When contact is made, when it briefly insinuates itself into our minds, we encounter its vague uncertainty as something to be feared, and, accordingly, something to be avoided. But, as illustrated with the enabling frames of previous chapters, what if all people were able to access an ongoing relationship to my-death in ways that enhance their lives? What if all of us were to approach my-death as something to embrace rather than to shun? And if we were to do that, what might be some of the ways of promoting such relationships so they become widely acceptable and generally accessible in our lives?

Death Awareness Movement

In the 1960s and early 1970s, two influential books on death, focusing on quite different areas, managed to turn a general disinterest in the topic into a focus of considerable public interest. First, Elizabeth Kubler-Ross's seminal book *On Death and Dying*[2] highlighted the need to understand the psychological processes that occur around dying and bereavement. Then, a few years later, Ernest Becker's *The Denial of Death*[3] highlighted the broader social implications of ignoring death. Whether these and other books generated the interest or whether they connected to something that was already stirring in the public consciousness is a moot point. But probably the willingness to turn and face personal mortality resonated with something that was happening on a wider front. More recently, Lucy Bregman (2003) in her book on the death awareness movement, highlighted how, in the past forty years, we are "no longer stuck in silence and denial of death," and much of this change can be tracked to the ground swell of public interest in shifting perspectives on death.[4] She identified how both traditional religions (such as Christianity and Buddhism) and various modern iterations of spirituality have contributed in complex ways to this change. The following brief overview will concentrate on three aspects of this movement: self-help networks, the rise of professional and educational associations, and the introduction of public health approaches.[5]

Let's first consider the role of self-help networks in promoting death awareness. In 2004, a Swiss sociologist, Bernard Crettaz, organized the first Death Café—or "Café Mortel"—in Neuchâtel. He was concerned about the struggles people were having in talking about death, and he envisioned Death Cafés as informal occasions in which people met up to talk openly about all aspects of death. From this small beginning, Death Cafés spread into many countries thereby turning them into a truly global self-help movement. Meetings are typically two to three hours in length, set in informal settings, and supplied with plenty of coffee and cake. Client–therapist relationships are consciously discouraged in favor of equal sharing and respectful listening. Those turning up share a broad range of experiences, ideas, and stories related to death. The topics discussed are also wide-ranging and typically include ways of responding to the death of loved ones, preferences regarding the process of dying, how one's own funeral will be conducted, and philosophical discussions on the meaning of death.[6]

In his book on Death Cafés, Jack Fong (2017) linked their proliferation to the way baby-boomers are now entering phases in their life where concerns about dying have become more pressing. He characterized the Cafés as essentially a social movement in which meetings provided a focal point for common communities of interest. He described attendees as

> *preparing for death early in life, whether viscerally from inspirational sentiments provided by fellow attendees, or from deep within their own experiences with personal loss, in hopes of living their days with deeper purpose. As Death Café events are now systematically accessible around the world, Death Cafés can be seen as a vital organ of civil society, a new iteration of a death system beyond the hospital.*[7]

In his closing chapter, Fong praised Cafés for the way they enable attendees to "decolonize" their relationship to death from standard forms of understanding and for the way they discourage handing over "sovereignty" of death to experts.[8]

The four characters in this book capture some of the spirit of what Death Cafés aim to achieve. In their dialogues, they connect with each other at regular times to talk about death and what it means to them, and, as in the Cafés, their discussions have ranged widely, with each character forging his or her own pathway. However, these conversations differ from those in the Cafés in one important way: their primary focus is on my-death. While the conversations of Café attendees might traverse aspects of my-death, they concentrate mainly on either other-death issues—such as bereavement and preparing loved ones for dying—or other-death applications to personal mortality—such as fear of death and planning for one's own funeral.

Brenda scuffled out from her shower wearing a floral dressing-gown and with her hair wrapped in a towel. She found Mandy in the kitchen baking muffins. "Ah, that smells nice."

"Comfort food, I suppose," responded Mandy as she greased the muffin tins. "Brenda, I've been meaning to say, I think our conversations about death have opened up so many things for me in ways I never expected. I am grateful for the way you've both listened and shared."

"Hmm, they've been important for me as well," said Brenda dipping a finger in the bowl to sample the muffin mixture. "See, while at work we talk a lot about death and dying, seldom would I get a chance to talk specifically about my own death. Up until we started talking about it, I had no idea how confused and avoidant I'd been."

"Huh, you avoidant? What about me?"

"Yeah, I think it's been an unusual journey for all of us," commented Brenda. "And, speaking personally, the switch into my new way of thinking about death has made a big difference."

"In what way?" asked Mandy as she spooned the mixture into the little cups in the muffin tin.

"Oh, in lots of ways. At work I feel more confident talking to patients about how they view dying. Also, I think it's helped me clarify what's important in life and what I want out of it. I also feel calmer and less worried about the little things."

"Heck, that's quite a number of changes," said Mandy lifting up the tray and nodding for Brenda to open the oven door. She slipped the tray in, closed the oven, then leaned on the counter with her back to the oven. "Don't you think it would be good to encourage others to develop how they think about their own death?"

"Hmm, I don't think I'm quite ready for that," stated Brenda, "but if I was, I reckon it would require strategies for getting people to talk more regularly and openly about their own deaths. It needs to be seen as a normal topic for conversation. And there's just so much working against that. You used to say it yourself: it's morbid and depressing to talk about your own death, and should definitely not be encouraged."

"Yeah, I remember, but I changed, and so can other people. We just need to find opportunities for them to sit down with each other and talk through possibilities. We, for example, have come up with four quite different possibilities. Couldn't these become the base for having conversations?"

Death Cafés are one example out of a range of self-help activities marking a general shift in willingness to think and speak about death. An increasing range of self-help books, such as Stephen Levine's (2010) *Healing into Life and Death* and Sallie Tisdale's (2018) *Advice for Future Corpses (and Those Who Love Them)*, offer practical guidance on managing death issues including responding to bereavement, thinking about death, and preparing to die.[9] Supplementing these, the internet has opened up a range of communication options which include discussion forums, such as the UK-based website DyingMatters.org and the Canadian-based TalkDeath.com, and websites with videos of people talking about death, such as those on the Catholic site

ArtofDyingWell.org and the US-based site DeathOverDinner.org. A further type of resource are death awareness computer applications, or "apps," such as those that provide death messages at regular intervals (e.g., WeCroak) and those which use population data to provide personalized estimates of time left to live (e.g., DeathClock and DeathCalculator). However, as with the Death Cafés, these resources tend to focus more on other-death issues by configuring dying as an absence from a continuing world rather than as the threat of total annihilation.

In contrast to the grassroots activities of self-help networks, the death awareness movement also gained momentum through the emergence of specialist health professionals who, like Brenda, worked in places specifically designed for the care of the dying. In 1967, in a residential suburb of London, Dame Cicely Saunders set up the first hospice, St. Christopher's, which then became a model for similar early hospices in Connecticut and California before spreading to many countries around the world.[10] Saunders could see how the hospital wards, where most people died, were becoming increasingly clinical and cure-oriented and, as such, were failing to provide the sort of holistic care appropriate for people who are dying and their families. Alongside the building of hospices came the emergence of specialist medical and nursing professionals who worked in them and who soon developed their own professional networks that, over time, consolidated into professional associations such as the American National Hospice and Palliative Care Organization, the European Association for Palliative Care, and the International Psychosocial Oncology Society. As time moved on, and the holistic nature of working with the dying was more understood, professionals working in dying spaces diversified to include physiotherapists, occupational therapists, and those specifically focused on mental well-being, such as counselors and psychotherapists.

The professionalization of places for dying drove demand for training programs for the specialist professionals who worked with people at the end of life. Initially this took the form of on-the-job training which, over time, led to the development of educational programs supplying an increasing range of specialist qualifications (usually at a postgraduate level) offered by universities and some independent educational providers such as the US-based Association for Death Education and Counseling and the Australian-based Centre of Palliative Care. On the positive side, such programs have led to steady improvements in the range of practices and the quality of care for those who are dying.[11] Also, as a spin-off from postgraduate learning, they have fostered a wide variety of end-of-life research activities. On the less positive side, the professionalization of dying spaces has encouraged perceptions that engaging with the dying requires advanced levels of specialist knowledge and professional expertise. This perception has the potential to isolate these spaces from other healthcare environments, such as hospital staff, and from other parts of the community. We will look again at this and other aspects of health professional training in the next section.

Another branch of the death awareness movement to consider concerns a more recent application of public health principles to promoting stronger engagement with death and dying across the whole of society. Donald Acheson's (1988) elegant definition of public health described it as "the art and science of preventing disease, prolonging life and promoting health through the organized efforts of society."[12] The phrases "art and science" and "organized efforts" are critical in recognizing the importance of trying to change things at the level of whole populations. However, when it comes to death awareness, the term "prolonging life" seems somewhat incongruous; that is, until one looks a little closer at what might be intended by "promoting health." Health promotion is the branch of public health concerned with implementing changes within communities and broader society which lead to positive improvements in personal and social well-being. Much of health promotion has been influenced by the World Health Organization's (1988) Ottawa Charter, which envisaged such change as requiring multipronged initiatives that encompassed changes for the individual, for communities, for society, and for government policy.[13]

A key figure in recognizing the potential of public health in promoting death awareness has been the English sociologist, Allan Kellehear.[14] In his book *Compassionate Cities*, he lays out what a public health approach to dying might look like, making particular use of the applied strategies of health promotion and community empowerment. He contended that if we do not find a way of promoting community involvement in end-of-life care, then

> *this queue of professionals at the door of our homes and servicing our identities will see no end. Without community involvement, professional involvement must become a rationalization and poor substitute for the multidimensional relationships that any one person enjoyed before encountering the local health service. The social and economic costs in permitting this "professionalization" of death to continue are unimaginable.*[15]

Kellehear viewed the professionalization of dying spaces as creating obstacles to the empowerment of communities to determine how they would choose end of life to take place. In its stead, he lays out a long-term program for engaging communities and empowering those around to take an active role in determining how environments for the dying are configured and how people around them engage.[16]

While Kellehear's primary interest was in end-of-life contexts, his application of health promotion principles could be used to instill a stronger my-death presence into broader death awareness initiatives and to promote rich and diverse conversations about people's relationships to my-death. I would envisage this getting under way in the form of four interlocked phases: reviewing, empowering, planning, and acting. The first phase, reviewing, involves procedures for auditing the extent and quality of my-death engagement in particular death awareness activities. This would entail, for example, recording the proportion of time people in Death Cafés discuss my-death or the extent to which nursing training programs include discussions of my-death in their teaching on death and dying. The second phase, empowering, would use health promotion practices in bringing people together to discuss how they would like my-death engagement to occur in their communities. Open meetings would assist in identifying a small group of like-minded community members interested in change. The third phase, planning, would engage this group in designing a range of small initiatives for promoting discussion on my-death. For example, they might opt for a series of community presentations or public meetings. Responses to these would further inform the development of their plan. The fourth phase, action, would involve implementing their plan and seeking the involvement of other stakeholders (such as local authorities, hospices, and training institutions) in longer term attempts to improve my-death engagement.

Unfortunately, as we approach the end of this book, little space remains for further discussion of how to apply public health principles to my-death engagement. While Kellehear and others have made use of such principles in promoting death awareness in general, applications to my-death engagement are yet to be formulated, implemented, and tested.

End-of-Life Care

The provision of special places for the dying, and the professionals who work in them, has intersected with many of the discussions in this book. This is unavoidable because end-of-life care is, arguably, one of the most intensively researched areas in death studies. However, as repeatedly noted, the primary orientation of this research has focused squarely on other-death awareness. When my-death awareness is discussed, it tends to be only indirectly or inadvertently seen as relevant. Given the sheer volume of studies in this area, I now intend to shift attention onto questioning what has been learned about relationships with my-death from people who work with the dying.

> After getting dressed Brenda placed two buttered muffins on a plate then strolled into the living room, where she found Leo sprawled out on the couch playing games on his mobile phone.
>
> "Hi, Leo. I see your study's going well." She smiled, offering him a muffin before sitting down in the armchair.
>
> Leo smiled as he put his phone down and stated, "I don't know how you cope working day-in, day-out with the dying."
>
> "Hmm, it can be stressful some days, but we have a good team, and we look out for each other; constantly checking out that things are okay . . . I mean, that things are emotionally okay. We also make sure we debrief after tricky conversations and have regular supervision sessions."
>
> "Even so, if it was me seeing people pop-off all the time, I'd be looking out for less demanding jobs like being a politician or an air-traffic controller."
>
> "Hah, that's right," laughed Brenda. "But you need to remember, those who work with the dying see it more as a vocation than a career; for us, it's more than a job. We believe we're making a real difference for the people we see and for society as a whole."
>
> "But can you really see it as a job? I mean, dying is everyone's business. No one has a monopoly on what it means to die and how to handle it."

Most research into end-of-life care has taken the form of either surveys using standardized questionnaires or in-depth interviews with small sets of key professionals or their patients—usually ten to thirty participants—focusing on various aspects of their experience of the dying process. The topics studied have included the emotional impacts on staff, the nature of good and not-so-good deaths, and communication challenges in working with those who are dying.[17] For example, one area of interest has been the effects of constant exposure to the dying and its potential to impact negatively on staff in the form of death anxiety, job burnout, and compassion fatigue.[18] In a national survey of American oncology specialists, Deborah Whippen and George Canellos (1991) recorded 56 percent of their sample reporting burnout.[19] But, surprisingly, in a systematic review of studies on rates of burnout among palliative care professionals, Sandra Martins-Pereira and colleagues (2011) found overall that they were no higher than burnout rates for health professionals in other contexts.[20] Lisa Quinn-Lee and colleagues (2014) clarified this further by surveying 290 hospice social workers using measures of death anxiety and burnout. Their findings suggested that burnout was more closely linked to high workloads and insufficient support rather than the nature of their work.[21] This was backed up by Noemi Sansó and colleagues (2015) who asked 387 palliative care professionals in Spain to complete surveys on self-care and death aware-ness and found those with stronger self-care and stronger death awareness were less likely to experience negative effects such as burnout. In both studies the likelihood of burnout appeared to be mitigated by both strong mutual sup-port between staff and their willingness to seek meaning from their exposures to death. Similar results on the importance of meaning-making were found for doctors (Zambrano et al., 2013), for hospital nurses (Johansson and Lindahl, 2011), and for palliative care nurses (Ablett et al., 2007).[22]

These studies raise questions as to the forms of meaning-making which might be occurring. It suggests that many of those regularly exposed to dying are processing issues at a fundamental level, at a level where the spiritual and existential dimensions of my-death are being considered. Hayley Pessin and colleagues (2015) searched out research studies on the existential impacts on end-of-life care professionals. They managed to find eighteen relevant studies in which the existential distress experienced had both positive and negative outcomes, including those related to "one's own life experiences and ultimate mortality."[23] In one of the studies they reviewed, a study by Isabelle DeArmond (2013), seventeen hospice professionals in the United States were asked about aspects of personal growth associated with their work, and she identified five main elements which included opportunities for reflection, personal integra-tion of experiences, and a sense of connection with the life of the spirit. Of particular interest was the way her participants described integrating their experiences of other people dying into a larger reality by plugging into

> *a sense of interconnectedness with all human beings and a sense of connection to something bigger. They share the experience of the dying person and some-times the connection remains alive after their death.*[24]

Many of her informants described how working with the dying had strength-ened their appreciation of both life and spirituality and had reduced their death anxiety.

Similar negative and positive outcomes have been found with end-of-life care professionals in other countries.[25] For example, Wallace Chan and colleagues (2016) interviewed twenty-two palliative care professionals in Hong Kong and asked them to describe how they coped with the emotional and existential challenges they experienced in their work.[26] Their participants described how their work shattered many of their assumptions about death, and, to cope, they saw the need to address these existential issues by revaluing life priorities and goals and engaging in a "search for the meaning of suffering and death." In a similar study involving of Portuguese nurses, Vitor Parola and colleagues (2018) interviewed nine participants and, out of the five themes identified, one theme focused on how thinking about my-death makes

> one conscious of the ephemeral nature of life, inviting reflection, personal development, and the incorporation of changes in the way of thinking, being, and living life.[27]

In a study in the United States more specifically focused on the meaning of my-death, Rachel Rodenbach and colleagues (2016) interviewed thirty-three health professionals working with people dying from cancer about their perspectives on my-death. While all their informants recognized their own death as inevitable, they varied in the extent to which they felt at peace with their mortality. They divided these into three groups: a small group who reported full acceptance of my-death, another small group who did not accept their mortality and preferred not to think about it, and the largest group who reported accepting my-death conceptually but not existentially. They referred to this as "conditional acceptance" and commented that

> [w]hile they currently felt comfortable with their mortality, they acknowledged not knowing themselves fully enough to anticipate how they would react when faced with serious illness in the future. At this point in their lives, they occupied themselves with more immediate concerns such as career or family, and worries about death, when present, tended to be at the back of their minds.[28]

On this basis, they advocated an openness to discussing my-death as an important ingredient in communicating with the dying.

To sum this up, professionals who specialize in working with the dying tend to develop an appreciation of the process of dying, and this impacts on their understanding of their own death. But their work is demanding, and many struggle with more pressing challenges, such as the stress and the workload. Despite this, the preceding studies suggest that the meaning of my-death is, at least, part of the action and appears to contribute to positive experiences and to working effectively with the dying. This, then, raises the question of the extent to which my-death awareness is being included in the education and training of end-of-life care professionals.

Leo had polished off his muffin and was thinking about paying Stan a visit. "Okay, Brenda, when you were training, how were you originally prepared for talking with people about their own death?"

"In my palliative nurse training we didn't spend much time talking about our own deaths. Plenty about the process of dying, family issues, bereavement . . . handling our own feelings about patients dying . . . but I can't recall any teaching about my own death."

"That's a pity. It would've been good for trainees to have an opportunity to think and talk about it." Leo glanced across at Brenda with a mischievous expression. "Imagine in a teaching session if the four of us turned up and each took turns to explain our take on mortality. That would get everyone thinking."

"Yeah, yeah, that would be good. But not very practical. Besides, trainees would need some way of preparing for such a discussion."

"Well, just like what happens in study at my university, they could achieve that through some form of reflective writing exercise. Perhaps the teacher could ask them to write down their thoughts about their own death, or maybe keep some sort of journal on the topic."

Brenda smiled and nodded. "Hmm, and after that, a few weeks later, ask them to talk about it in class. And they could be given some written summaries of our different views which could stimulate ideas or provide the material for discussion. I can see how, with careful encouragement, and in a safe class environment, it could help trainees begin to explore what their own deaths mean to them."

"But you know what," exclaimed Leo, "it's not just palliative care nurses; the medical specialists who work with the dying would also benefit from this. I read somewhere that most people don't die at home, or in hospices, but die in hospitals. So shouldn't it be anyone who works in a hospital who is encouraged to think through how they view their own death?"

"Yes, good point," agreed Brenda. "There are some palliative care specialists working in hospitals, but most people aren't specialists; they're ordinary doctors, ordinary nurses, ordinary social workers . . . they're the ones who have most contact with the dying; they're the ones who would benefit most from such discussions."

"So how could they access such learning?"

"I guess it means introducing opportunities to reflect on one's own death into their basic training—such a big undertaking. Perhaps in their undergraduate programs, when death and dying is discussed, they could reserve part of their teaching sessions for discussing their own deaths."

Leo's point about where people die was backed up in a study by Joanna Broad and colleagues (2013), in which they brought together place-of-death data from forty-five countries and found that more than half (54 percent) died in hospitals, twelve percent died in residential aged care facilities, and around a third (32 percent) in other locations including homes.[29] Interestingly, they noted that despite widespread preference for dying at home, most deaths (more than two-thirds) occurred in institutions. The dominance of institutional environments reinforces Leo's queries regarding wider my-death education for health professionals.

My-death education could take a variety of forms. As already suggested, one option is to provide safe contexts in which open discussion on my-death can take place. Susann Strang and colleagues (2014) in Sweden invited nurses in daily contact with cancer patients to attend five sessions of group reflection where they discussed existential issues associated with death. They recorded and analyzed the reflection sessions and were able to identify a range of communication skills that their participants had found helpful including "being present and accommodating" and "being sensitive and confirming."[30] Rob Houtepen and David Hendrikx (2003) in a similar study looked at the challenges of communicating about existential issues and stated that

> [o]ur analysis shows that it takes a 'fine-tuned antenna' from nurses to determine these existential questions, which are often put indirectly and in a variety of forms.[31]

Their work highlighted the practice elements of working in this area and suggested the possibility of developing training based around the simulation of conversations about my-death. The role-playing of sensitive conversations with patients is a common teaching method in both nursing and medicine, and it has been used in training end-of-life professionals in conversations with dying patients and their families.[32] Such role playing could also be a safe and useful tool in helping those involved with the people at end of life to become practiced in talking about my-death.

Research and Scholarship

During the course of writing this book I spent six weeks in England at the University of York attached to their Department Health Science. In my first week there I contacted someone involved in death research who informed me that, in two days, downstairs in the same building, they were hosting an international conference called "Death and Culture II."[33] Intrigued by the coincidence, I asked if I might join in, and, for two days, I listened to speakers from many locations around the world presenting their research on death. What struck me about these presentations, and about conversations during breaks, was the absence of discussion on the nature and meaning of my-death. Plenty of discussion focused on rituals of dying, bereavement practices, and media and literary depictions. but these were nearly all oriented around death as understood as other-death. I wondered if this was simply the result of the focus on culture, but, since then, I have spoken with other death scholars who commented that an interest in my-death was unusual. I found this curious and wonder if it is something to do with the unspeakable nature of the topic which discourages interest and whether this has allowed the study of my-death to become dwarfed by an overwhelming focus on other-death.

The academic field of death studies has expanded rapidly in the past twenty years both in terms of the number of research publications and their breadth of coverage. Lectures on death are now commonplace in undergraduate teaching in sociology, anthropology, cultural studies, health studies, and even psychology. Research teams and units focused on death have been popping up in many locations around the world.[34] The range of different methods used to study death has also widened to include the highly objective methods (such as biological and experimental studies), highly subjective methods (such as lived experience interview studies), context-specific methods (such as ethnographic studies), and historical and theoretical scholarship. However, despite this accelerating interest in death, the narrower focus on how we think and engage with my-death has, on the whole, attracted only piecemeal attention.

Kate Woodthorpe (2011), in her discussion of research methods, makes the point that death is a topic "from which *no one* is exempt."[35] In other words, we are all insiders when it comes to the study of death. Indeed, I would take Woodthorpe's claim one step further and argue that not only is the narrower focus on my-death a topic from which no one is exempt but also that its importance permeates every stage of life and every aspect of how we engage with what it means to be alive. For this reason, and in line with other commentators,[36] research focused on my-death, by its very nature, places the personal experiences and perspectives of the researcher right at the center of what is being studied.

Leo let himself in through Stan's back door and found him polishing his military medals on the kitchen table.

"Ah Leo, come and look at this," said Stan beckoning him over to sit opposite. "Look at these medals. How do you think I managed to get all these?"

"They look impressive Stan," said Leo running his hands over the insignias. "But what's going to happen to them when you pass on?"

"Hmm, I thought I might leave a couple to you," he said, studying Leo's reaction.

"Oh, Stan, I'd so like that, I really would." Leo paused to inspect each one. "Ah, but Stan, what I've really come to talk about . . . well, me and Brenda we're thinking about ways we might share our various views on death with other people. You know, we've been talking about it among the four of us, and we've all benefited, so we thought others might benefit, too. For them it could become a normal and acceptable part of their lives. Just imagine. How could we make that happen?"

"Hmm, you know there's one thing which always makes a difference when you're setting out into new territories, and that's research. Before venturing into the unknown you need to investigate as best you can what the new terrain will involve. We did heaps of research before taking off into space and plenty of research before transplanting hearts."

"Okay, but besides Heidegger's work, I don't know anyone who's seriously researched their own death."

"Me neither, but there must be ways we can improve our understanding of this area, and just because it's tricky and elusive, that's no excuse for not trying to find ways forward."

"So, Stan, what would you like to see researched?"

"Well, I think among ourselves we've managed to come up with a number of different and interesting ways of thinking about our deaths which have strengthened our relationships with it in our lives. So what I'd like to know, first off, is what it means for people to live in these differently framed relationships."

"You mean that we track people with different ways of thinking and work out which is best?"

"Well, I don't expect one to be better than the other; just different. Nonetheless, one perspective may suit certain people more than others." Stan paused to think of examples. "Perhaps a more anxious person might benefit from a strong belief in the afterlife . . . and a more intellectual person might prefer, like you, a more structured approach. I dunno . . . perhaps it doesn't work that way, and we'll find people choose their perspectives for quite random reasons."

"Thanks for seeing me as more intellectual. I'll remember that," laughed Leo. "You know, I wonder if there are other possible ways of thinking about one's own death. We've come up with four; maybe there's even better ones we've never thought about."

"Maybe, but . . . but we have an even more fundamental question to tackle. The default position that most people accept is not thinking about their own death until just before they die. Is that okay? Or are there advantages thinking through your perspective much earlier?"

"Hmm, we could interview a bunch of people who have shifted from not thinking to thinking about their own death and ask them how things have changed since making that shift."

Stan smiled and nodded his agreement. "Yes, or we could take on an even larger study measuring changes in quality of life both before and after they start thinking about it." He rubbed his hands together enthusiastically. "Oh, there's so much we could do if we had enough time and money."

"And we could evaluate different strategies for promoting awareness of one's own death. Strategies like discussion sessions and training for nurses and doctors."

"Yes, there is much that's crying out for investigation."

So far, we have ventured into many areas of death studies research and scholarship, including what is on offer in the main disciplines of philosophy, psychology, social sciences, and health studies. Each chapter has attempted to glean from these dispersed literatures ideas relevant to my-death. At this point it is worth reflecting back on where interest in my-death has been concentrated and to make some general observations about where my-death studies might head in the future.

Let's start with philosophy and its related disciplines of theology and ethics. At the core of each of the four enabling frames introduced earlier is a philosophical discussion on how to both think and speak about my-death. Leo explored sources in ontology, Stan drew on ideas from existential writers, Mandy referenced sources from theology and the philosophy of religion, and Brenda ventured into postmodern thinking. Further philosophical enquiry could help in deepening our understanding of these four enabling frames and in exploring other possibilities. Alongside these enquiries is the question of language. What are we doing when we use these frames to speak about my-death? What are the rhetorical elements—such as metaphor and metonymy—and how effectively are they being deployed?

Psychology is a complex discipline with many very different subspecialties stretching from the realism of cognitive and behavioral psychology to the constructivism of existential and postmodern psychology. In research psychology, the strongest areas of interest include questionnaire studies on our fear of death, development studies on children's conceptions of death, and, more recently, experimental studies on terror management theory. In clinical psychology and related applied psy sciences, interest has focused on existential issues associated with my-death, but efforts have been spasmodic and concentrated mostly on issues related to other-death rather than my-death. As suggested by Leo and Stan, psychology could examine more closely the meanings and life-impacts of my-death and the way such awareness connects with other processes such as life span development and identity formation.

In the social sciences, particularly sociology, anthropology, and media and cultural studies, considerable effort has gone into studying customary practices around death, including the nature of funeral and bereavement rituals and depictions of death in literature, film, and other media. However, most these efforts have focused on the death of other people and very little has focused on the social and cultural dynamics of my-death. Many of the same forms of research could be redirected into exploring issues associated with my-death, such as the role of my-death imagery in media and literary depictions, the relationship between my-death engagement and cultural practices, and the contribution of my-death awareness to social processes such as social cohesion and social change.

Research interest in health studies has mainly focused on end-of-life care issues such as the lived experience of those who are dying and ways of improving health professional responses. As signaled by Stan, research and scholarship specifically targeting my-death engagement could contribute positively to research in the future, but, as with the other disciplines, the dominant focus has been on other-death more than my-death. Nonetheless, there are some important questions that could be asked regarding my-death engagement. Do increases in my-death awareness earlier in life assist with the end-of-life phase? What are the health and mental health impacts of using enabling frames to assist in my-death engagement? What strategies would be effective in promoting my-death awareness in the whole population?

Notes

1. From Epicurus, "Letter to Menoeceus," *Epicurus: The Extant Remains* (Oxford: Oxford University Press, 1926), pp. 83–93.
2. E. Kübler-Ross, *On Death and Dying* (New York: Scribner, 1969).
3. E. Becker, *The Denial of Death* (New York: Free Press, 2007, 1973).
4. L. Bregman, *Death and Dying, Spirituality and Religions: A Study of the Death Awareness Movement* (New York: Peter Lang, 2003). She makes this claim on p. 3.
5. An overview of the movement is provided by K. Doka in "The death awareness movement," in C. Bryant, ed., *Handbook of Death and Dying* (Thousand Oaks, CA: Sage, 2003) pp. 50–56.
6. The global spread of Death Cafés is detailed by Jack Fong, *The Death Café Movement* (Cham, Switzerland: Springer, 2017). The movement's spread in the United States and the range of topics discussed is detailed by L. Miles and C. Corr in "Death Café: What is it and what we can learn from it," *Omega: Journal of Death and Dying* (75:2, 151–65, 2017).
7. J. Fong, *The Death Café Movement*, p. 29.
8. Ibid., p. 259. Similar high praise for Death Cafés can be found in Jules Morgan, "Celebrating life in a Death Café," *The Lancet Neurology* (16:9, 690, 2017) and R. Nelson, "Discussing death over coffee and cake," *American Journal of Nursing* (117:2, 18–19, 2017).
9. S. Levine, *Healing into Life and Death* (New York: Knopf Doubleday, 2010) and S. Tisdale, *Advice for Future Corpses (and Those Who Love Them): A Practical Perspective on Death and Dying* (New York: Touchstone, 2018).
10. See Linda Camobell, "History of the hospice movement," *Cancer Nursing* (9:6, 333–38, 1986).

11. An overview of professional training for those working with those at the end of life is provided by P. Gillan, P. van der Riet, and S. Jeong in "End of life care education, past and present," *Nurse Education Today* (34, 331–42, 2014).

12. From the report by D. Acheson, *Public Health in England* (London: HMSO, 1988), the definition which was later adopted by the World Health Organization.

13. World Health Organization, *The Ottawa Charter for Health Promotion* (Geneva: WHO, 1988).

14. See the evolution of his approach in A. Kellehear and D. O'Connor, "Health-promoting palliative care," *Critical Public Health* (18:1, 111–15, 2008) and his "Death education as a public health issue," in J. Stillion and T. Attig, eds., *Death, Dying, and Bereavement* (New York: Springer, 2014) pp. 221–33.

15. A. Kellehear, *Compassionate Cities: Public Health and End-of-Life Care* (London: Taylor & Francis, 2012) p. ix.

16. The use of the Ottawa Charter in developing health-promoting palliative care is reviewed by L. Sallnow et al. in "The impact of a new public health approach to end-of-life care," *Palliative Medicine* (30:3, 200–11, 2016), and further discussed by J. Rosenberg and P. Yates in "Health promotion in palliative care," *Critical Public Health* (20:2, 201–10, 2010).

17. On "good deaths" see J. Mak and M. Clinton, "Promoting a good death," *Nursing Ethics* (6:2, 97–106, 1999).

18. See the survey by S. Slocum-Gori et al. in "Understanding compassion satisfaction, compassion fatigue and burnout," *Palliative Medicine* (27:2, 172–78, 2013).

19. See the survey of oncologists by D. Whippen and G. Canellos in "Burnout syndrome in the practice of oncology," *Journal of Clinical Oncology* (9:10, 1916–20, 1991).

20. See the review by S. Martins Pereira, A. Fonseca, and A. Carvalho in "Burnout in palliative care," *Nursing Ethics* (18:3, 317–26, 2011).

21. See L. Quinn-Lee, L. Olson-McBride, and A. Unterberger, "Burnout and death anxiety in hospice social workers," *Journal of Social Work in End-of-Life & Palliative Care* (10:3, 219–39, 2014).

22. For doctors, see S. Zambrano, A. Chur-Hansen, and G. Crawford, "The experiences, coping mechanisms, and impact of death and dying on palliative medicine specialists," *Palliative and Supportive Care* (12:4, 309–16, 2013); for hospital nurses, see K. Johansson and B. Lindahl, "Moving between rooms: Moving between life and death," *Journal of Clinical Nursing* (21:13/14, 2034–43, 2012); and for palliative care nurses, see J. Ablett and R. Jones, "Resilience and well-being in palliative care staff," *Psycho-Oncology* (16:8, 733–40, 2007).

23. See H. Pessin et al., "Existential distress among healthcare providers caring for patients at the end of life," *Current Opinion in Supportive and Palliative Care* (9:1, 77–86, 2015).

24. I. DeArmond, "The psychological experience of hospice workers during encounters with death," *Omega: Journal of Death and Dying* (66:4, 281–99, 2013) p. 290.

25. For example, see an exploration of the experiences of hospice nurses in Taiwan by H.-L. Wu and D. Volkner in "Living with death and dying," *Oncology Nursing Forum* (36:5 578–84, 2009); with Canadian palliative care providers by P. Boston and B.

Mount in "The caregiver's perspective on existential and spiritual distress in palliative care," *Journal of Pain and Symptom Management* (32:1, 13–26, 2006); and with
hospice nurses in Denmark by L. Ingebretsen and M. Sagbakken in "Hospice nurses'
emotional challenges in their encounters with the dying," *International Journal of
Qualitative Studies on Health and Wellbeing* (11:1, 31170, 2016).

26. W. Chan et al., "Impact of death work on self," *Health & Social Work* (41:1,
33–41, 2016).

27. V. Parola et al., "Caring in palliative care," *Journal of Hospice & Palliative Nursing*
(20:2, 180–6, 2018) p. 183. Also relevant to the transformational potential of working
with the dying is R. Mota Vargas et al., "The transformation process for palliative care
professionals," *Palliative Medicine* (30:2, 161–70, 2016).

28. R. Rodenbach et al., "Relationships between personal attitudes about death and communication with terminally ill patients," *Patient Education and Counseling* (99:3,
356–63, 2016) p. 358.

29. J. Broad et al., "Where do people die?," *International Journal of Public Health* (58:2,
257–67, 2013).

30. See S. Strang et al., "Communication about existential issues with patients close to
death," *Psycho-Oncology* (23:5, 562–68, 2014).

31. R. Houtepen and D. Hendrikx, "Nurses and the virtues of dealing with existential
questions in terminal palliative care," *Nursing Ethics* (10:4, 377, 2003) p. 377.

32. See P. Gillan, S. Jeong, and P. van der Riet, "End of life care simulation," *Nurse
Education Today* (34, 706–14, 2014).

33. This was the second conference run by the Death and Culture Network (DaCNet)
based at the University of York.

34. Examples of units and networks in the United Kingdom include Death and Culture
Network (DaCNet) based at the University of York, the Centre for Death and Life
Studies at Durham University, Centre of Death & Society at the University of Bath,
and the Sheffield Death Group in Sociology.

35. K. Woodthorpe, "Researching death," *International Journal of Social Research
Methodology* (14:2, 99–109, 2011) p. 100.

36. For a review of the types of research and methodologies, see E. Borgstrom and J. Ellis,
"Introduction: Researching death, dying and bereavement," *Mortality* (22:2, 93–104,
2017), and the case for including one's own subjectivity in death research is made by
R. Visser in "'Doing death': Reflecting on the researcher's subjectivity and emotions,"
Death Studies (41:1, 6–13, 2017).

Conclusion

I found this book difficult to write and did not anticipate it being so challenging. Many a time I found myself staring at the computer screen wondering how on earth to gain a foothold on such an elusive subject. Several hours on I would still be struggling with what to say. Indeed, what can you say about my-death other than it is inevitable and unthinkable?

These times forced me to reflect on the wisdom of taking on this topic in the first place. What attracted me to such an abstruse and impenetrable topic? Was it my immersion forty years ago in Heidegger's ideas on death? Was it working as a clinical psychologist with clients who were grappling with existential dilemmas? Was it my more recent interest in bringing existential concerns into the orbit of public health? Perhaps it was all these factors combined.

The book's main challenge focused on ways in which a relationship with my-death might, in the face of its unintelligibility, become a regular part of our daily lives. Solid barriers immediately presented themselves, not the least of which was the unspeakable nature of my-death and the knock-on fear and avoidance that follows from such uncertainty. Nonetheless, I was persuaded that engaging with mortality was, on balance, more beneficial than trying to ignore it. The main obstacle identified was the absence of ways of thinking and talking about my-death, and, to that end, discussion focused on a set of four devices, four "enabling frames," which were proposed as conceptual vehicles for engaging with personal mortality. Each frame was built around a central idea, such as an afterlife, and crisscrossed by rhetorical supports such as recurring metaphors and associative (metonymic) linkages.

The merits of each of these four frames—essential structures, passionate suffusion, point-of-transition, and self-generative process—were explored separately before being compared together. In the process of contrasting their strengths it became clear that different people are likely to prefer different frames in line with their varying temperaments, cultural exposures, and religious affiliations. For this reason, the future utility of such frames will depend on efforts to both renew current frames and further develop alternative frames. This would provide us with a menu of options for engaging with my-death which could, in turn, form the basis for my-death awareness initiatives such as self-help networks and educational strategies.

While on the journey of writing this book I was grateful for the company of the four characters whose conversations sprinkled discussion with liveliness and complexity. It would be, admittedly, very unlikely for four such characters to choose to simultaneously engage in changing how they think about my-death. Crisis periods like these are rare events and unlikely to occur together. So, while their conversations were contrived, they unfolded in a way that highlighted the possibilities for my-death engagement across different ages and stages of life, across different life circumstances, and across varying levels of exposure to other-death. I want to finish by saying a brief goodbye to the four characters who have accompanied us on this journey.

Mandy carried a glass of fruit juice and a piece of cake over to the table under the shade of the ginkgo tree at the corner of the yard. The midsummer sun was baking the concrete pavers, and she had to walk quickly to avoid burning her bare feet. She sighed as she reached the shade and sat down to gaze out at the shimmering haze.

She thought back over the events of the past year: so many discussions, so many changes. . . . And now things are changing again. Brenda has decided to leave. She'll miss her. And Leo has been awarded a scholarship to study postgraduate biomedical science in another city. While she was proud of his achievement, she worried about how he will cope without her . . . or, maybe, how she will cope without him.

Brenda sauntered out in her dressing gown and slippers carrying a bottle of water. "Mandy, what a hot morning."

"Yes, scorching. It's going to be really hot by midday." She glanced up at Brenda and beckoned her to sit down. "How's your packing going?"

"Oh, that won't take long. I haven't hoarded much."

"Very sensible. So what's your new apartment like?"

"It's on the second floor overlooking a park. It's closer to the city and includes a covered carpark."

"I knew your stay was always going to be temporary, but, I must say, I've really enjoyed having you around."

"Yes Mandy . . . it's been such an important time for me. . . . I plummeted down into such a dark place, and, with your support, I managed to crawl out and clamber up to a much better spot. Thank you for all you've done and all you've shared."

"No, no. It's me who should be grateful. Up until my mystical encounter I was lost. I was fighting with shadows; growling at others, including you, whenever there was any talk of death. Then, through our discussions, I found myself in a new space."

"Don't worry. I understand why it was so hard: your husband dying, Leo's fascination with death, your concerns for his welfare . . . I quite understand."

Leo sauntered out using both hands to shade his eyes from the bright sunshine. "Ah, you two, talking about death again?" He joined them sitting at the table.

Brenda smiled across at him. "Leo, I heard you're leaving?"

"Yep. Time to move on. Time the old girl learns to live without me; she'll have to face it someday."

"Go on," laughed Mandy. "The old girl's more than ready for her cub to leave the pride."

Leo looked up and noticed Stan edging sideways through the hole in the fence then hobbling across the lawn to join them in the shade.

Stan sat down and wiped the sweat away from his forehead. "Heard all your voices and decided I didn't want to miss out." He paused to catch his breath. "And, through the grapevine, a little bird told me both Leo and Brenda are leaving."

"Yes, that's right," said Mandy. "We won't be able to carry on our conversations about death anymore."

"Ah, but haven't we done well on that front," declared Brenda.

Stan smiled. "Yes, that's true. I've certainly learned to appreciate life differently." He glanced at them each in turn. "And I've had some good news. I went for a checkup yesterday and the doctor's told me my heart's improving. He reminded me it was still damaged and I would have to be careful, but as long as I eat well and take my medication, he doesn't see why I couldn't live another ten years."

"Oh Stan, that's wonderful news," said Mandy. "So no more sitting on death's doorstep."

"But the heart attack has already worked its magic. I plan to continue thinking about death and talking about it with anyone who will listen."

"I'm going to miss that," said Brenda. "I'm leaving early tomorrow, so I mightn't see you again before I leave. I could. . . ."

"I tell you what," interrupted Leo. "Why don't we try to stay in touch and update each other on our interactions with death?"

"Hmm, not a bad idea," Brenda concurred. "We could email each other, or do it live through the computer."

"Yes, or I could set up a Facebook page," suggested Leo. "A closed page available only to us, and every now and then we could write a post updating how things are progressing."

"I'm not so good interneting and posting and all that," muttered Stan.

"Don't worry," said Mandy. "I can help you there. We could do it together."

"Great, so that's what we'll do," declared Leo.

The four companions sat in silence listening to the chorus of cicadas in the trees and watching the breeze fluttering through the leaves.

Brenda sighed. "It feels like we're all venturing out . . . setting out into new adventures."

Bibliography

Abdollahi A, Henthorn C, Pyszczynski T. Experimental peace psychology: Priming consensus mitigates aggression against outgroups under mortality salience. *Behav Sci Terrorism Pol Aggression*. 2010;2:30–37.

Ablett JR, Jones J. Resilience and well-being in palliative care staff: A qualitative study of hospice nurses' experience of work. *Psycho-Oncology*. 2007;16(8):733–40.

Acheson D. *Public Health in England: The Report of the Committee of Inquiry into the Future Development of the Public Health Function*. London: HMSO; 1988.

Adams PJ. Switching to a social approach to addiction: Implications for theory and practice. *Int J Ment Health Ad*. 2015;14:86–94.

Adams PJ. *Moral Jeopardy: The Risks of Accepting Money from Tobacco, Alcohol and Gambling Industries*. Cambridge: Cambridge University Press; 2016.

Adams PJ. Oscillating imbalances: Responding to the existentials in major life transitions. *J Soc Work Prac*. 2017;31(3):323–36.

Adams PJ. *Navigating Everyday Life: Exploring the Tension Between Finitude and Transcendence*. Lanham, MA: Lexington Books; 2018.

Aday RH. Belief in afterlife and death anxiety: Correlates and comparisons. *OMEGA J Death Dying*. 1985;15(1):67–75.

Adorno FP. Against posthuman ideology: Aesthetics and finitude of the individual. *Res Anthro Aesthet*. 2010;57–58:344–54.

Ahn E, Shin DW, Choi JY, et al. The impact of awareness of terminal illness on quality of death and care decision making: A prospective nationwide survey of bereaved family members of advanced cancer patients. *Psycho-Oncology*. 2013;22(12):2771–78.

Almeder RF. *Death and Personal Survival: The Evidence for Life After Death*. Lanham MA: Rowman & Littlefield; 1992.

Almond PC. *Afterlife: A History of Life after Death*. London: I. B. Tauris; 2016.

Anthony S. *The Child's Discovery of Death: A Study in Child Psychology*. Abingdon Oxon: Routledge; 2013 (1940).

Ardelt M. Wisdom, religiousity, purpose in life, and death attitudes of aging adults. In Tomer A, Eliason GT, Wong P, ed. *Existential and Spiritual Issues in Death Attitudes*. Mahwah, NJ: Lawrence Erlbaum, 2013:139–58.

Arendt H. *The Human Condition*. Chicago, IL: University of Chicago Press; 1958.

Aries P. *Western Attitiudes Toward Death: From the Middle Ages to the Present*. Trans: P M. Ranum. Baltimore, MD: Johns Hopkins University Press; 1974.

Ariès, P. *The Hour of Our Death* (1st American ed.). New York: Knopf; 1981.

Arndt J, Vess M. Tales from existential oceans: Terror management theory and how the awareness of our mortality affects us all. *Soc Pers Psychol Compass*. 2008;2(2):909–28.

Arnett J. Reckless behavior in adolescence: A developmental perspective. *Dev Rev*. 1992;12(4):339–73.

Augustine K. Near-death experiences are hallucinations. In Martin M, Augustine, K, eds. *The Myth of an Afterlife: The Case Against Life After Death*. Lanham, MD: Rowman & Littlefield; 2015:529–70.

Austin JL. *How to Do Things with Words*. Cambridge, MA: Harvard University Press; 1975 (1962).

Baker LR. Death and the afterlife. In Wainwright WJ, ed. *The Oxford Hanbook of Philosophy of Religion*. Oxford: Oxford Univesity Press; 2007:366–91.

Balk DE, Corr CA. Adolescents, developmental tasks and encounters with death and bereavement. In Corr CA, Balk DE, eds. *Handbook of Adolescent Death and Bereavement*. New York: Springer; 2004:3–24.

Barad K. Posthumanist performativity: Toward an understanding of how matter comes to matter. *Signs: J Women Culture Society*. 2003;28(3):801–31.

Barbour IG. *Religion and Science*. San Francisco, CA: HarperCollins; 2013.

Bassett JF, Connelly JN. Terror management and reactions to undocumented immigrants: Mortality salience increases aversion to culturally dissimilar others. *J Soc Psych*. 2011;151(2):117–20.

Becker E. *The Denial of Death*. New York: Free Press; 2007 (1973).

Belshaw C. *Annihilation: The Sense and Significance of Death*. Stockfield, UK: Acumen; 2009.

Benore ER, Park CL. Death-specific religious beliefs and bereavement: Belief in an afterlife and continued attachment. *Int J Psychol Religion*. 2004;14(1):1–22.

Bergson HL. *Time and Free Will: An Essay in the Immediate Data of Consciousness*. Trans: Pogson FL. New York: Macmillan; 1910.

Bering J. Intuitive conceptions of dead agents' minds: The natural foundations of afterlife beliefs as phenomenological boundary. *J Cognition Culture*. 2002;2(4):263–308.

Bhattacharya P. Is there science behind the near-death experience: Does human consciousness survive after death? *Ann Trop Med Public Health*. 2013;6(2):151–65.

Bishop KW. *American Zombie Gothic: The Rise and Fall (and Rise) of the Walking Dead in Popular Culture*. Jefferson, NC: McFarland; 2011.

Blass T, ed. *Obedience to Authority: Current Perspectives on the Milgram Paradigm*. London: Psychology Press; 1999.

Blattner W. Is Heidegger a representationalist? *Philos Top*. 1999;27(2):179–204.

Bluebond-Langner M. *The Private Worlds of Dying Children*. Princeton, NJ: Princeton University Press; 1980 (1978).

Booth WC. *The Rhetoric of Rhetoric: The Quest for Effective Communication*. Malden, MA: Blackwell Publishing; 2004.

Borah P. Conceptual issues in framing theory: A systematic examination of a decade's literature. *J Communication*. 2011;61(2):246–63.

Borgstrom E, Ellis J. Introduction: Researching death, dying and bereavement. *Mortality*. 2017;22(2):93–104.

Boston P, Bruce A, Schreiber R. Existential suffering in the palliative care setting: An integrated literature review. *J Pain Sympt Manag*. 2011;41(3):604–18.

Boston PH, Mount BM. The caregiver's perspective on existential and spiritual distress in palliative care. *J Pain Sympt Manag*. 2006;32(1):13–26.

Brain JL. *The Last Taboo: Sex and the Fear of Death*. Garden City, NY: Anchor/ Doubleday; 1979.

Bregman L. *Death and Dying, Spirituality and Religions: A Study of the Death Awareness Movement*. New York: Peter Lang; 2003.

Brent SB, Speece MW. "Adult" conceptualization of irreversibility: Implications for the development of the concept of death. *Death Stud.* 1993;17(3):203–24.

Broad JB, Gott M, Kim H, Boyd M, Chen H, Connolly MJ. Where do people die? An international comparison of the percentage of deaths occurring in hospital and residential aged care settings in 45 populations, using published and available statistics. *Int J Public Health.* 2013;58(2):257–67.

Bronfenbrenner U. *The Ecology of Human Development.* Cambridge, MA: Harvard University Press; 1979.

Bronfenbrenner U, ed. *Making Human Beings Human: Bioecological Perspectives on Human Development.* Thousand Oaks, CA: Sage; 2004.

Brooks P, Gewirtz PD. *Law's Stories: Narrative and Rhetoric in the Law.* New Haven, CT: Yale University Press; 1996.

Bucke RM. *Cosmic Consciousness: A Study in the Evolution of the Human Mind.* New York: Dutton & Co; 1923 (1901).

Burke BL, Martens A, Faucher EH. Two decades of terror management theory: A meta-analysis of mortality salience research. *Pers Social Psychol Rev.* 2010;14(2):155–95.

Butler J. *Bodies That Matter: On the Discursive Limits of "Sex.* New York: Psychology Press; 1993.

Butler J. *Subjects of Desire: Hegelian Reflections in Twentieth-Century France.* New York: Columbia University Press; 2012.

Camobell L. History of the hospice movement. *Cancer Nurs.* 1986;9(6):333–38.

Cant R, Cooper S, Chung C, O'Connor M. The divided self: Near death experiences of resuscitated patients: A review of literature. *Int Emergency Nurs.* 2012;20(2):88–93.

Carpenter RH. *History as Rhetoric: Style, Narrative, and Persuasion.* Columbia: University of South Carolina Press; 1995.

Carr D, Sharp S. Do afterlife beliefs affect psychological adjustment to late-life spousal loss? *J Gerontology Ser B Psychol Sci Soc Sci.* 2014;69(1):103–12.

Ceci SJ, Bronfenbrenner U. On the demise of everyday memory: "The rumors of my death are much exaggerated" (Mark Twain). *Am Psychol.* 1991;46(1):27–31.

Chan WCH, Fong A, Wong KLI, Tse DMW, Lau KS, Chan LN. Impact of death work on self: Existential and emotional challenges and coping of palliative care professionals. *Health Soc Work.* 2016;41(1):33–41.

Chang C-Y. *Creativity and Taoism: A Study of Chinese Philosophy, Art and Poetry.* London: Wildwood House; 1963.

Chong D, Druckman JN. Framing Theory. *Ann Rev Pol Sci.* 2007;10(1):103–26.

Collett LJ, Lester D. The fear of death and the fear of dying. *J Psychol.* 1969;72(2): 179–81.

Combs J, Freedman G. *Narrative Therapy: The Social Construction of Preferred Realities.* New York: Norton & Co; 1996.

Corcoran PE. *Political Language and Rhetoric.* Brisbane: University of Queensland Press; 1979.

Cotton CR, Range LM. Children's death concepts: Relationship to cognitive functioning, age, experience with death, fear of death, and hopelessness. *J Clin Child Psychol.* 1990;19(2):123–27.

Cox M, Garrett E, Graham JA. Death in Disney films: Implications for children's understanding of death. *OMEGA J Death Dying.* 2005;50(4):267–80.

Cozzolino PJ. Death contemplation, growth, and defense: Converging evidence of dual-existential systems? *Psychol Inquiry.* 2006;17(4):278–87.

Cozzolino PJ, Blackie L, Meyers LS. Self-related consequences of death fear and death denial. *Death Stud.* 2014;38(6):418–22.

Dasgupta S. *Indian Idealism.* Cambridge: Cambridge University Press; 1963.

Dastur F. *Death: An Essay in Finitude.* Trans: Llewelyn J. London: Athlone; 1996.

De Quincey T. *Selected Essays on Rhetoric.* Carbondale: Southern Illinois University Press; 2010 (1897).

DeArmond IM. The psychological experience of hospice workers during encounters with death. *OMEGA J Death Dying.* 2013;66(4):281–99.

Depelteau F. Relational thinking: A critique of co-deterministic theories of structure and agency. *Sociol Theory.* 2008;26(1):51–73.

Deppman J. Dickinson, death, and the sublime. *Emily Dickinson J.* 2000;9(1):1–20.

Derrida J. *Aporias.* Trans: Dutoit T. Stanford, CA: Stanford University Press; 1993.

Derrida J. *Voice and Phenomenon: Introduction to the Problem of the Sign in Husserl's Phenomenology.* Trans: Lawlor L. Evanston, IL: Northwestern University Press; 2011.

Dickerson AB. *Kant on Representation and Objectivity.* Cambridge: Cambridge University Press; 2004.

Dickstein LS, Blatt SJ. Death concern, futurity, and anticipation. *J Consult Psychol.* 1966;30(1):11–17.

Dickstein LS. Attitudes toward death, anxiety, and social desirability. *OMEGA J Death Dying.* 1978;8(4):369–78.

Dirven R, PoringsR, eds. *Metaphor and Metonymy in Comparison and Contrast.* Berlin: Mouton de Gruyter; 2002.

Dixon P. *Rhetoric.* London: Methuen; 1971.

Doka KJ. the death awareness movement: Description, history and analysis. In Bryant CD, ed. *Handbook of Death and Dying, Volume 1: The Presence of Death.* Thousand Oaks, CA: Sage; 2003:50–56.

Downey AM. Relationship of religiosity to death anxiety of middle-aged males. *Psychol Rep.* 1984;54(3):811–22.

Dubois J, Edeline F, Klinkenberg J, Minguet P, Pine F, Trinon H. *A General Rhetoric.* Trans: Burrel P, Slotkin E. Baltimore, MD: John Hopkins University Press; 1981 (1970).

Durkheim E. *Suicide: A Study in Sociology.* Taylor & Francis, e-book; 2005 (1951).

Ellis L, Wahab EA. Religiosity and fear of death: A theory-oriented review of the empirical literature. *Rev Religious Res.* 2013;55(1):149–89.

Entman RM. *Projects of Power: Framing News, Public Opinion, and US Foreign Policy.* Chicago, IL: University of Chicago Press; 2004.

Eschleman A. The afterlife: Beyond belief. *Int J Philos Religion.* 2016;80(2):163–83.

Facco E, Agrillo C, Greyson B. Epistemological implications of near-death experiences and other non-ordinary mental expressions: Moving beyond the concept of altered state of consciousness. *Med Hypotheses.* 2015;85(1):85–93.

Field D, Copp G. Communication and awareness about dying in the 1990s. *Palliative Med.* 1999;13(6):459–68.

Firestone R, Catlett J. *Beyond Death Anxiety: Achieving Life-Affirming Death Awareness.* New York: Springer; 2009.

Flannelly KJ, Koenig HG, Ellison CG, Galek K, Krause N. Belief in life after death and mental health: Findings from a national survey. *J Nerv Ment Dis.* 2006;194(7):524–29.

Flores RF. The capacity to begin: Arendt's concept of "natality" (a humble tribute on the 40th anniversary of her death). *Threads.* 2015;3:80–87.

Florian V, Kravetz S. Fear of personal death: Attribution, structure, and relationship to religious belief. *J Pers Soc Psychol.* 1983;44:600–07.

Florian V, Mikulincer M. The impact of death-risk experiences and religiosity on the fear of personal death: The case of Israeli soldiers in Lebanon. *OMEGA J Death Dying.* 1993;26(2):101–11.

Florian V, Mikulincer M, Hirschberger G. An existentialist view on mortality salience effects: Personal hardiness, death-thought accessibility, and cultural worldview defence. *Brit J Soc Psychol.* 2001;40(3):437–53.

Fong J. *The Death Café Movement: Exploring the Horizons of Mortality.* Cham, Switzerland: Springer; 2017.

Frankl V. *The Doctor and the Soul: From Psychotherapy to Logotherapy.* New York: Knopf; 1952.

Freud S. *Reflections on War and Death.* Trans: Brill AA, Kuttner AB. New York: Moffat, Yard & Co; 1918.

Freund AM, Ritter JO. Midlife crisis: A debate. *Gerontology.* 2009;55(5):582–91.

Frie R. On the nature and meaning of human finitude. *Am J Psychoanalysis.* 2013;73:158–72.

Furedi F. *Culture of Fear Revisited: Risk-Taking and the Morality of Low Expectation, Fourth Edition.* London: Continuum; 2006.

Gallup G, Proctor W. *Adventures in Immortality: A Look Beyond the Threshold of Death.* New York: McGraw-Hill; 1982.

Gamson W, Modigliani A. Media discourse and public opinion on nuclear power: A constructionist approach. *Am J Sociol.* 1989;95(1):1–37.

Gardner S. Kant's practical postulates and the limits of the critical system. *Hegel Bull.* 2013;32(1–2):187–215.

Gavrilova TA. The problem of children's understanding of death. *Psychol Sci Educ.* 2009;4(online).

Gentner D, Stevens A, eds. *Mental Models.* New York: Lawrence Erlbaum; 1983.

Gergen KJ. *Relational Being: Beyond Self and Community.* Cary, NC: Oxford University Press, 2009.

Gertsman E. Pleyinge and peyntynge: Performing the dance of death. *Stud in Iconography.* 2006;27:1–43.

Ghosh S. *Hindu Concept of Life and Death: As Portrayed in Vedas, Brahmanas, Aranyakas, Upanisads.* New Delhi: Munshiram Manoharlal Publishers; 2002.

Gillan P, Jeong S, van der Riet PJ. End of life care simulation: A review of the literature. *Nurs Educ Today.* 2014;34:706–74.

Gillan P, van der Riet PJ, Jeong S. End of life care education, past and present: A review of the literature. *Nurs Educ Today.* 2014;34:331–42.

Gillies J, Neimeyer RA. Loss, Grief, and the search for significance: Toward a model of meaning reconstruction in bereavement. *J Constructivist Psychol.* 2006;19(1):31–65.

Glaser BG, Strauss AL. *Awareness of Dying.* New Brunswick: Aldine Transaction; 1966.

Gower PL. *Psychology of Fear.* New York: Nova Science; 2004.

Grant AM, Wade-Benzoni KA. The hot and cool of death awareness at work: Mortality cues, aging, and self-protective and prosocial motivations. *Acad Manag Rev.* 2009;34(4):600–32.

Greyson B. The Near-Death Experience Scale: Construction, reliability, and validity. *J Nerv Ment Dis.* 1983;171(6):369–75.

Greyson B. Reduced death threat in near-death experiencers. In Neimeyer RA, ed. *Death Anxiety Handbook: Research, Instrumentation, and Application*. London: Routledge; 2015:169–80.

Hacking I. *Representing and Intervening: Introductory Topics in the Philosophy of Natural Science*. Cambridge: Cambridge University Press; 1983.

Hankiss E. *Fears and Symbols: An Introduction to the Study of Western Civilization*. Budapest: CEU Press; 2001.

Hartshorne C. *Reality as Social Process: Studies in Metaphysics and Religion*. New York: Free Press; 1953.

Harvell LA, Nisbett GS, eds. *Denying Death: An Interdisciplinary Approach to Terror Management Theory*. New York: Routledge; 2016.

Hegel GWF. *Phenomenology of Spirit*. Trans Miller AV, Findlay JN. Oxford: Oxford University Press; 1977.

Hegel GWF. *Encyclopedia of the Philosophical Sciences in Basic Outline, Part 1, Science of Logic*. Trans: Brinkmann K, Dahlstrom KO. Cambridge: Cambridge University Press; 2015 (1825).

Heidegger M. *Being and Time*. Trans: Macquarrie J, Robinson E. Oxford: Basil Blackwell; 1973 (1927).

Heidegger M. *The Fundamental Concepts of Metaphysics: World, Finitude, Solitude*. Trans: McNeill W, Walker N. Bloomington: Indiana University Press; 2001 (1938).

Heidegger M. *Kant and the Problem of Metaphysics, Fifth Edition*. Trans: Taft R. Bloomington: Indiana University Press; 1997 (1929).

Heidegger M. The Thing. *Poetry, Language, Thought*. Trans: Hofstader A. New York: Harper & Row; 1971:161–84.

Heinämaa S. The many senses of death: Phenomenological insights into human death. In Hakola O, Heinämaa S, Pihlström S, ed. *Death and Mortality: For Individual to Communal Perspectives*. Helsinki: Helsinki Collegium for Advanced Studies; 2015:100–18.

Henriksen J-O. *Finitude and Theological Anthropology: An Interdisciplinary Exploration into Theological Dimensions of Finitude*. Leuven: Peeters; 2011.

Hesiod. *Hesiod: Theogony, Works and Days, Shield*. Trans: Athanassakis AN. Baltimore, MD: Johns Hopkins University Press; 2004.

Hodge KM. On imagining the afterlife. *J Cognition Culture*. 2011;11(3–4):367–89.

Hopkins M. *The Development of Children's Understanding of Death*. PhD Thesis. University of East Anglia; 2014.

Houtepen R, Hendrikx D. Nurses and the Virtues of dealing with existential questions in terminal palliative care. *Nurs Ethics*. 2003;10(4):377.

Howells K, Gould M, Field D. Fear of death and dying in medical students: Effects of clinical experience. *Med Educ*. 1986;20(6):502–06.

Husserl E. *Cartesian Meditations: An Introduction to Phenomenology*. Trans: Cairns D. Dordrecht: Kluwer Academic; 1999 (1901).

Ingebretsen LP, Sagbakken M. Hospice nurses' emotional challenges in their encounters with the dying. *Int J Qualitative Stud Health Well-Being*. 2016;11(1):31170.

Ireton SM. *An Ontological Study of Death: From Hegel to Heidegger*. Pittsburgh, PA: Duquesne University Press; 2007.

Irish DP, Lundquist KF, Nelsen VJ, eds. *Ethnic Variations in Dying, Death and Grief: Diversity in Universality*. Philadelphia, PA: Taylor & Francis; 2014.

James W. *The Varieties of Religious Experience*. New York: Longmans; 1902.

Janoff-Bulman R, Frantz CM. The impact of trauma on meaning: From meaningless world to meaningful life. In Power MJ, Brewin CR, eds. *The Transformation of Meaning in Psychological Therapies: Integrating Theory and Practice*. Hoboken, NJ: Wiley; 1997:91–106.

Jaques E. Death and the mid-life crisis. *Int J Psychoanalysis*. 1965;46(4):502–14.

Jay SM, Green V, Johnson S, Caldwell S, Nitschke R. Differences in Death concepts between children with cancer and physically healthy children. *J Clin Child Psychol*. 1987;16(4):301–06.

Johansson K, Lindahl B. Moving between rooms—moving between life and death: Nurses' experiences of caring for terminally ill patients in hospitals. *J Clin Nurs*. 2012;21(13–14):2034–43.

John J. Representationism, phenomenism, and the intuitive view. *Philos Topics*. 2005;33(1):159–84.

Jonas E, Fritsche I. Destined to die but not to wage war: How existential threat can contribute to escalation or de-escalation of violent intergroup conflict. *Am Psychol*. 2013;68(7):543–58.

Jong J, Ross R, Philip T, Chang S-H, Simons N, Halberstadt J. The religious correlates of death anxiety: A systematic review and meta-analysis. *Relig Brain Behav*. 2018;8(1):4–20.

Juhl J, Routledge C. Putting the terror in terror management theory: Evidence that the awareness of death does cause anxiety and undermine psychological well-being. *Curr Dir Psychol Sci*. 2016;25(2):99–103.

Kagan S. *Death*. New Haven, CT: Yale University Press; 2012.

Kant I. *Critique of Judgement*. Trans: Meredith JC. Oxford: Oxford University Press; 1952 (1892).

Kant I. *Critique of Practical Reason*. Trans: Gregor MJ. Cambridge: Cambridge University Press; 1997 (1788).

Kant I. *Critique of Pure Reason*. Trans: Guyer P, Wood AW. Cambridge: Cambridge University Press; 1998 (1787).

Kellehear A. On dying and human suffering. *Palliat Med*. 2009;23(5):388–397.

Kellehear A. *Compassionate Cities: Public Health and End-of-Life Care*. London: Taylor & Francis; 2012.

Kellehear A. Death Education as a public health issue. In Stillion JH, Attig T, eds. *Death, Dying, and Bereavement: Contemporary Perspectives, Institutions, and Practices*. New York: Springer; 2014:221–33.

Kellehear A, O'Connor D. Health-promoting palliative care: A practice example. *Crit Public Health*. 2008;18(1):111–15.

Kelly J. *The Great Mortality: An Intimate History of the Black Death*. New York: HarperCollins; 2006.

Kennedy GA. *A New History of Classical Rhetoric*. Princeton, NJ: Princeton University Press; 1994.

Kenyon BL. Current research in children's conceptions of death: A critical review. *OMEGA J Death Dying*. 2001;43(1): 63–91.

Kierkegaard S. *The Sickness Unto Death: A Christian Psychological Exposition of Edification and Awakening by Anti-Climacus*. Trans: Hannay A. London: Penguin Classics; 2004 (1849).

Kinsella M. Near-death experiences and networked spirituality: The emergence of an afterlife movement. *J Am Acad Religion*. 2017;85(1):168–98.

Knoblauch H, Schmied I, Schnettler B. Different kinds of near-death experience: A report on a survey of near-death experiences in Germany. *J Near-Death Stud*. 2001;20(1):15–29.

Koepke S, Denissen J. Dynamics of identity development and separation–individuation in parent–child relationships during adolescence and emerging adulthood: A conceptual integration. *Dev Rev*. 2012;32(1):67–88.

Kojève A. The idea of death in the philosophy of Hegel. In Keenan DK, ed. *Hegel and Contemporary Continental Philosophy*. Albany: State University of New York Press; 2004:27–75.

Kotter-Grühn D, Grühn D, Smith J. Predicting one's own death: The relationship between subjective and objective nearness to death in very old age. *Eur J Ageing*. 2010;7(4):293–300.

Krell DF. *Intimations of Mortality: Time, Truth, and Finitude in Heidegger's Thinking of Being*. University Park: Pennsylvania State University Press; 1986.

Kübler-Ross E. *On Death and Dying*. New York: Scribner; 1969.

Lakoff G. *Women, Fire, and Dangerous Things: What Categories Reveal About the Mind*. Chicago, IL: University of Chicago Press; 1987.

Landau MJ. Kosloff S, Schmeichel BJ. Imbuing everyday actions with meaning in response to existential threat. *Self Identity*. 2011;10(1):64–76.

Lazar A. Fear of personal death as a predictor of motivation for religious behavior. *Rev Relig Res*. 2006;48(2):179–89.

Lee RLM. Modernity, mortality and re-enchantment: The death taboo revisited. *Sociology*. 2008;42(4):745–59.

Lester D. The Collett-Lester Fear of Death Scale. In Neimeyer RA, ed. *Death Anxiety Handbook: Research, Instrumentation, and Application*. London: Routledge; 2015:45–60.

Levinas E. *God, Death, and Time*. Trans: Bergo B. Stanford CA: Stanford University Press; 2000.

Levine S. *Healing into Life and Death*. New York: Knopf Doubleday; 2010.

Lewis AM. Terror management theory applied clinically: Implications for existential-integrative psychotherapy. *Death Stud*. 2014;38(6):412–17.

Leymore V. *Hidden Myth: Structure and Symbolism in Advertising*. London: Heinemann; 1975.

Lizza JP. *Persons, Humanity and the Definition of Death*. Baltimore, MD: John Hopkins University Press; 2005.

López A, del Rosario M. "An infinite task at the heart of finitude": Jean-Luc Nancy on community and history. *CR: New Centennial Rev*. 2017;17(3):21–42.

Loxley J. *Performativity*. London: Routledge; 2006.

Lynette R. *The Grim Reaper*. Farmington Hills, MI: KidHaven Press; 2010.

Lyng S. Existential transcendence in late modernity: Edgework and hermeneutic reflexivity. *Human Stud*. 2012;35(3):401–14.

Lyng S. Sociology at the edge: Social theory and voluntary risk taking. In Lyng S, ed. *Edgework: The Sociology of Risk Taking*. New York: Routledge; 2005:17–49.

MacCormac ER. Religious metaphors: Mediators between biological and cultural evolution that generate transcendent meaning. *Zygon*. 1983;18:45–65.

MacCormac ER. *Metaphor and Myth in Science and Religion*. North Carolina: Duke University Press; 1976.

Macintosh JJ. The impossibility of Kantian immortality. *Dialogue*. 1980;19(2):219–234.

Magid O. Heidegger on human finitude: Beginning at the end. *Eur J Philos.* 2017;25(3):657–76.

Magni KG. The fear of death: An exploratory study of its nature and its correlates. In Godin A, ed. *Death and Presence: The Psychology of Death and Afterlife.* Brussels: Lumen Vitae; 1972:125–38.

Mahon MM. Death in the lives of children. In Talwar V, Harris PL, Schleifer M, eds. *Children's Understanding of Death: From Biological to Religious Conceptions.* Cambridge: Cambridge University Press; 2011:61–97.

Mak JMH, Clinton M. Promoting a good death: An agenda for outcomes research—a review of the literature. *Nurs Ethics.* 1999;6(2):97–106.

Markus A. *Beyond Finitude: God's Transcendence and the Meaning of Life.* Frankfurt: Peter Lang; 2004.

Martin M, Augustine K, eds. *The Myth of an Afterlife: The Case Against Life After Death.* Lanham, MD: Rowman & Littlefield; 2015.

Martins Pereira S, Fonseca AM, Carvalho AS. Burnout in palliative care: A systematic review. *Nurs Ethics.* 2011;18(3):317–26.

Matheson B. Practical identity. In Nagasawa Y, Matheson B, eds. *The Palgrave Handbook of the Afterlife.* London: Palgrave Macmillan; 2017:391–411.

McClain-Jacobson C, Rosenfeld B, Kosinski A, Pessin H, Cimino JE, Breitbart W. Belief in an afterlife, spiritual well-being and end-of-life despair in patients with advanced cancer. *Gen Hosp Psychiat.* 2004;26(6):484–86.

McIntosh S, Leverette M, eds. *Zombie Culture: Autopsies of the Living Dead.* Lanham, MD: Scarecrow Press; 2008.

McManus R. *Death in a Global Age.* Basingstoke, UK: Palgrave Macmillan; 2012.

Merton T. *Zen and the Birds of Appetite.* New York: New Directions; 1968.

Mikulincer M, Florian V. The complex mulifaceted nature of the fear of personal death. In Tomer A, Eliason GT, Wong PTP, eds. *Existential and Spiritual Issues in Death Attitudes.* New York: Laurence Erlbaum; 2013:29–64.

Mikulincer M, Florian V, Hirschberger G. The existential function of close relationships: Introducing death into the science of love. *Pers Soc Psychol Rev.* 2003;7(1):20–40.

Miles L, Corr CA. Death Cafe: What is it and what we can learn from it. *OMEGA J Death Dying.* 2017;75(2):151–65.

Moraglia G. On facing death: Views of some prominent psychologists. *J Humanist Psychol.* 2004;44(3):337–57.

Moreman CM. *Beyond the Threshold: Afterlife Beliefs and Experiences in World Religions* (2nd ed.). Lanham, MD: Rowman & Littlefield; 2017 (2008).

Morgan J. Celebrating life in a Death Cafe. *Lancet Neurology.* 2017;16(9):690.

Mota Vargas R, Mahtani-Chugani V, Pallero MS, Jiménez BR, Domínguez RC, Alonso VR. The transformation process for palliative care professionals: The metamorphosis, a qualitative research study. *Palliat Med.* 2016;30(2):161–70.

Moustakas C. *Phenomenological Research Methods.* Thousand Oaks, CA: Sage; 1994.

Nagasawa Y, Matheson B, eds. *The Palgrave Handbook of the Afterlife.* London: Palgrave Macmillan; 2017.

Nagy M. The child's theories concerning death. *J Genet Psychol.* 1948;73:3–27.

Nancy J-L. *Being Singular Plural.* Stanford, CA: Stanford University Press; 2000.

Nancy J-L. *A Finite Thinking.* Stanford, CA: Stanford University Press; 2003.

Neimeyer RA, ed. *Death Anxiety Handbook: Research, Instrumentation, and Application.* London: Routledge; 2015.

Neimeyer RA, Wittkowski J, Moser RP. Psychological research on death attitudes: An overview and evaluation. *Death Stud.* 2004;28(4):309–40.

Nelson R. Discussing death over coffee and cake: The emergence of the Death Café. *Am J Nurs.* 2017;117(2):18–19.

Nichols T. *Death and Afterlife: A Theological Introduction.* Grand Rapids, MI: Brazos Press; 2010.

Noppe IC, Noppe LD. Adolescent experiences with death: Letting go of immortality. *J Ment Health Counseling.* 2004;26(2):146–67.

Noppe LD, Noppe IC. Ambiguity in adolescent understandings of death. In Corr CA, Balk DE, eds. *Handbook of Adolescent Death and Bereavement.* New York: Springer; 2004:25–42.

Nouel G. Construction of meaning in the face of mortality. In Tomer A, Eliason GT, Wong PTP, eds. *Existential and Spiritual Issues in Death Attitudes.* New York: Laurence Erlbaum; 2013:235–55.

O'Byrne A. *Natality and Finitude.* Bloomington, IN: Indiana University Press; 2010.

Oberst JL. *Heidegger on Language and Death: The Intrinsic Connection in Human Existence.* London: Continuum; 2009.

Orbach I. Existentialism and suicide. In Tomer A, Eliason GT, Wong P, eds. *Existential and Spiritual Issues in Death Attitudes.* New York: Laurence Erlbaum; 2001:281–316.

Osborne JW. An existential perspective on death anxiety, retirement, and related research problems. *Can J Aging.* 2017;36(2):246–55.

Österlind J, Hansebo G, Andersson J, Ternestedt BM, Hellström I. A discourse of silence: Professional carers reasoning about death and dying in nursing homes. *Ageing Soc.* 2011;31(4):529–44.

Panagiotaki G, Nobes G, Ashraf A, Aubby H. British and Pakistani children's understanding of death: Cultural and developmental influences. *Brit J Devel Psychol.* 2015;33(1):31–44.

Parola V, Coelho A, Sandgren A, Fernandes O, Apóstolo J. Caring in palliative care: A phenomenological study of nurses' lived experiences. *J Hospice Palliat Nurs.* 2018;20(2):180–86.

Pattison G. *Heidegger on Death: A Critical Theological Essay.* Surrey, UK: Ashgate; 2013.

Pereira V, Faísca L, de Sá-Saraiva R. Immortality of the soul as an intuitive idea: Towards a psychological explanation of the origins of afterlife beliefs. *J Cognition Culture.* 2012;12(1–2):101–27.

Perelman C. *The New Rhetoric and the Humanities: Essays on Rhetoric and Its Implications.* Dortrecht, Holland: D. Reidel; 1979.

Perelman C. *The Realm of Rhetoric.* Trans:Kluback W. Notre Dame, IN: University of Notre Dame Press, 1982.

Perera M, Padmasekara G, Belanti J. Prevalence of near-death experiences in Australia. *J Near-Death Stud.* 2005;24:109–16.

Pessin H, Fenn N, Hendriksen E, DeRosa AP, Applebaum A. Existential distress among healthcare providers caring for patients at the end of life. *Curr Opinion Supportive Palliat Care.* 2015;9(1):77–86.

Pihlström S. *Death and Finitude: Toward a Pragmatic Transcendental Anthropology of Human Limits and Mortality.* Lanham, MD: Lexington Books, 2016.

Poling DA, Hupp JM. Death sentences: A content analysis of children's death literature. *J Genet Psychol.* 2008;169(2):165–76.

Powell C, Dépelteau F. *Conceptualizing Relational Sociology: Ontological and Theoretical Issues.* New York: Palgrave Macmillan; 2013.

Pyszczynski T, Greenberg J, Solomon S. A Dual-process model of defense against conscious and unconscious death-related thoughts: An extension of terror management theory. *Psychol Rev.* 1999;106(4):835–45.

Pyszczynski T, Greenberg J, Solomon S, Maxfield M. On the unique psychological import of the human awareness of mortality: Theme and variations. *Psychol Inquiry.* 2006;17(4):328–56.

Quinn-Lee L, Olson-McBride L, Unterberger A. Burnout and death anxiety in hospice social workers. *J Soc Work End-of-Life Palliat Care.* 2014;10(3):219–39.

Razinsky L. *Freud, Psychoanalysis and Death.* Cambridge: Cambridge University Press; 2013.

Reid JD, Willis SL. Middle age: New thoughts, new directions. In Willis SL, Reid JD, eds. *Life in the Middle: Psychological and Social Development in Middle Age.* San Diego, CA: Academic Press; 1999:276–80.

Ricoeur P. *Fallible Man: Philosophy of the Will.* Trans: Kelbley CA. New York: Fordham University Press; 1986.

Ring K. *Life after Death: A Scientific Investigation of the near-Death Experience.* New York: Coward, McCann and Geoghenan; 1980.

Rilke RM. "Letter to Countess Margot Sizzo-Noris-Crouy, Epiphany," In Macy J, Barrows A, ed, trans. *A Year with Rilke: Daily Readings from the Best of Rainer Maria Rilke.* New York: HarperCollins, 1923.

Robert M, Tradii L. Do we deny death? I. A genealogy of death denial. *Mortality.* 2019;23(3): 247–60.

Rockmore T. Heidegger and representationalism. *Hist Philos Quart.* 1996;13(3):363–74.

Rodenbach RA, Rodenbach KE, Tejani MA, Epstein RM. Relationships between personal attitudes about death and communication with terminally ill patients: How oncology clinicians grapple with mortality. *Patient Educ Counseling.* 2016;99(3): 356–63.

Rorty R. *Consequences of Pragmatism (Essays 1972–80).* Minneapolis: University of Minnesota Press; 1991.

Rosen SJ, ed. *Ultimate Journey: Death and Dying in the World's Major Religions.* Westport, CT: Praeger; 2008.

Rosenberg JP, Yates PM. Health promotion in palliative care: The case for conceptual congruence. *Crit Public Health.* 2010;20(2):201–10.

Rosenberg JF. *Thinking Clearly About Death.* Indianapolis, IN: Hackett Publishing; 1998.

Ross LM, Pollio HR. Metaphors of death: A thematic analysis of personal meanings. *OMEGA J Death Dying.* 1991;23(4):291–307.

Russell JB. *A History of Heaven: The Singing Silence.* Princeton, NJ: Princeton University Press; 1998.

Sallnow L, Richardson H, Murray SA, Kellehear A. The impact of a new public health approach to end-of-life care: A systematic review. *Palliat Med.* 2016;30(3):200–11.

Sartre J-P. *Being and Nothingness.* Trans: Barnes HE. New York: Washington Square Press; 1992 (1943).

Schön DA. Generative metaphor: A perspective on problem-setting in social policy. In Ortony A, ed. *Metaphor and Thought.* Cambridge: Cambridge University Press; 1993:137–63.

Schumacher BN. *Death and Mortality in Contemporary Philosophy*. Trans: Miller MJ. Cambridge: Cambridge University Press; 2010.

Schutz A. *The Phenomenology of the Social World*. Evanston, IL: Northwestern University Press; 1967.

Sedgwick E, Frank A. *Touching Feeling: Affect, Pedagogy, Performativity*. Durham, NC: Duke University Press; 2003.

Segal A. *Life after Death: A History of the Afterlife in Western Religion*. New York: Doubleday; 2010.

Sexton J. The semantics of death and dying: Metaphor and mortality. *ETC Rev Gen Semantics*. 1997;54(3):333–45.

Silbereisen RK, Lerner RM. *Approaches to Positive Youth Development*. Los Angeles: Sage; 2007.

Sill JS. Disengagement reconsidered: Awareness of finitude. *Gerontologist*. 1980; 20(4):457–62.

Simons HW. *Rhetoric in the Human Sciences*. London: Sage; 1989.

Sinclair S. Impact of death and dying on the personal lives and practices of palliative and hospice care professionals. *Can Med Ass J*. 2011;183(2):180–87.

Slaughter V, Griffiths M. Death understanding and fear of death in young children. *Clin Child Psychol Psychiat*. 2007;12(4):525–35.

Sleutjes A, Moreira-Almeida A, Greyson B. Almost 40 years investigating near-death experiences: An overview of mainstream scientific journals. *J Nerv Ment Dis*. 2014;202(11):833–36.

Slocum-Gori S, Hemsworth D, Chan WWY, Carson A, Kazanjian A. Understanding compassion satisfaction, compassion fatigue and burnout: A survey of the hospice palliative care workforce. *Palliat Med*. 2013;27(2):172–78.

Sluga HD. *Heidegger's Crisis: Philosophy and Politics in Nazi Germany*. Cambridge, MA: Harvard University Press; 1995.

Sluss DM, Ashforth BE. Relational identity and identification: Defining ourselves through work relationships. *Acad Manag Rev*. 2007;32(1):9–32.

Solomon RC, Higgins KM. *The Age of German Idealism*. London: Routledge; 2003.

Soskice JM. *Metaphor and Religious Language*. Oxford: Clarendon Press; 1985.

Spall B, Read S, Chantry D. Metaphor: Exploring its origins and therapeutic use in death, dying and bereavement. *Int J Palliat Nurs*. 2001;7(7):345–53.

Spilka B, Pelligrini R, Dailey K. Religion, American values and death perspective. *Sociolog Symp*. 1968;1:57–66.

Stace WT. *Mysticism and Philosophy*. London: Macmillan; 1961.

Stack S, Gundlach J, Reeves JL. The heavy metal subculture and suicide. *Suicide Life-Threatening Behav*. 1994;24(1):15–23.

Staudinger UM, Bluck S. A view on midlife development from life-span theory. In Lachman ME, ed. *Handbook of Midlife Development*. Hoboken, NJ: Wiley; 2001:3–39.

Stets JE, Burke PJ. Identity theory and social identity theory. *Soc Psychol Quart*. 2000;63(3):224–37.

Stokols D. The social ecological paradigm of wellness promotion. In Jamner MS, Stokols D, eds. *Promoting Human Wellness: New Frontiers for Research, Practice, and Policy*. Berkeley: University of California Press; 2000:21–37.

Strang S, Henoch I, Danielson E, Browall M, Melin-Johansson C. Communication about existential issues with patients close to death: Nurses' reflections on content, process and meaning. *Psycho-Oncology*. 2014;23(5):562–68.

Stryker S. Traditional symbolic interactionism, role theory, and structural symbolic interactionism: The road to identity theory. In Turner JH, ed. *Handbook of Sociological Theory*. Boston, MA: Springer, 2001:211–31.

Sullivan D, Greenberg J, eds. *Death in Classic and Contemporary Film: Fade to Black*. New York: Palgrave Macmillan; 2013.

Szasz T. *Fatal Freedom: The Ethics and Politics of Suicide*. Syracuse, NY: Syracuse University Press; 2002, 1999.

Tacey D. *Religion as Metaphor: Beyond Literal Belief*. Abingdon, UK: Routledge; 2017.

Taminiaux J. *Dialectic and Difference: Finitude in Modern Thought*. Trans: Crease R, Decker JT. New York: Humanities Press; 1985.

Thau M. *Consciousness and Cognition*. Oxford: Oxford University Press; 2002.

Thomas SE. *What Is the New Rhetoric?* Newcastle, UK: Cambridge Scholars Publishing; 2007.

Thompson E. Empathy and consciousness. *J Consciousness Stud*. 2001;8(6–7):1–32.

Tillich P. *Systematic Theology*. London: Nisbet & Co.; 1953.

Tisdale S. *Advice for Future Corpses (and Those Who Love Them): A Practical Perspective on Death and Dying*. New York: Touchstone; 2018.

Tomer A, Eliason GT, Wong PTP, eds. *Existential and Spiritual Issues in Death Attitudes*. Mahwah, NJ: Lawrence Erlbaum, 2013.

Townsend C. *Art and Death*. London: I. B. Tauris; 2008.

Twenge J M, Sherman RA, Exline JJ, Grubbs JB. Declines in american adults' religious participation and beliefs, 1972–2014. *Sage Open*. 2016:6(1):2158244016638133.

Tye M. *Consciousness Revisited: Materialism Without Phenomenal Concepts*. Cambridge, MA: MIT Press; 2011.

Tye M. Representationalist theories of consciousness. In Beckermann A, McLaughlin B, Walter S, ed. *The Oxford Handbook of Philosophy of Mind*. Oxford: Oxford University Press; 2009:253–67.

US Department of Health and Human Services. *The Health Consequences of Smoking— 50 Years of Progress: A Report of the Surgeon General*. Atlanta, GA: US Department of Health and Human Services, CDCP, NCCDPHP, OSH; 2014.

Underhill E. *Mysticism: A Study in the Nature and Development of Man's Spiritual Consciousness*. London: Methuen; 1911.

Vail KE, Juhl J, Arndt J, Vess M, Routledge C, Rutjens BT. When death is good for life: Considering the positive trajectories of terror management. *Pers Soc Psychol Rev*. 2012;16(4):303–29.

Vallega AA. *Sense and Finitude: Encounters at the Limits of Language, Art, and the Political*. Albany: State University of New York Press, 2009.

van den Berg C, Soeters J. Self-perceptions of soldiers under threat: A field study of the influence of death threat on soldiers. *Milit Psychol*. 2009;21(sup2):S16–30.

Vickers B. *In Defence of Rhetoric*. Oxford: Clarendon Press; 1988.

Visser RC. "Doing death": Reflecting on the researcher's subjectivity and emotions. *Death Stud*. 2017;41(1):6–13.

Weiss D. What will remain when we are gone? finitude and generation identity in the second half of life. *Psychol Aging*. 2014;29(3):554–62.

Wendell L. *Encounters with Death: A Compendium of Anthropomorphic Personifications of Death from Historical to Present Day Phenomenon*. New Orleans, LA: Westgate; 1996.

Whippen DA, Canellos GP. Burnout syndrome in the practice of oncology: Results of a random survey of 1,000 oncologists. *J Clin Oncology*. 1991;9(10):1916–20.

White CJ. *Time and Death: Heidegger's Analysis of Finitude.* Aldershot, UK: Ashgate; 2005.

White G. *Talking About Spirituality in Health Care Practice: A Resource for the Multi-Professional Health Care Team.* London: Jessica Kingsley; 2006.

Whitehead AN. *Modes of Thought.* New York: Free Press; 1968 (1938).

Whitehead AN. *Process and Reality.* New York: Free Press; 2010 (1929).

Widera-Wysoczańska A. Everyday awareness of death: A qualitative investigation. *J Humanist Psychol.* 1999;39(3):73–92.

Wildman WJ. *Effing the Ineffable: Existential Mumblings at the Limits of Language.* Albany: State University of New York Press; 2018.

Wink P, Scott J. Does religiousness buffer against the fear of death and dying in late adulthood? Findings from a longitudinal study. *J Gerontology.* 2005;60b(4):207–14.

Winterowd ER. *Rhetoric: A Synthesis.* New York: Holt, Rinehart & Winstone; 1968.

Woodthorpe K. Researching death: Methodological reflections on the management of critical distance. *Int J Soc Res Method.* 2011;14(2):99–109.

Wordsworth W. *Ode: Intimations of Immortality from Recollections of Early Childhood.* Boston, MA: D. Lothrop & Co.; 1884.

World Health Organisation. *The Ottawa Charter for Health Promotion.* Geneva: WHO; 1988.

Wright JE. *The Early History of Heaven.* Oxford: Oxford University Press; 2002.

Wu H-L, Volker DL. Living with death and dying: The experience of Taiwanese hospice nurses. *Oncology Nurs Forum.* 2009;36(5):578–84.

Yalom ID, Lieberman M. Bereavement and heightened existential awareness. *Psychiatry.* 1991;54(4):334–45.

Yalom ID. Staring at the Sun: Overcoming the Terror of Death. *Humanist Psychol.* 2008;36(3–4):283–97.

Yalom ID. *When Nietzsche Wept: A Novel of Obsession.* New York: Basic Books; 1992.

Yalom ID. *Staring at the Sun: Overcoming the Terror of Death.* San Francisco, CA: Jossey-Bass; 2010.

Yang SC, Chen S-F. Content analysis of free-response narratives to personal meanings of death among Chinese children and adolescents. *Death Stud.* 2006;30(3):217–41.

Yoon S, Lam TH. The illusion of righteousness: Corporate social responsibility practices of the alcohol industry. *BMC Public Health.* 2013;13:630.

Zambrano SC, Chur-Hansen A, Crawford GB. The experiences, coping mechanisms, and impact of death and dying on palliative medicine specialists. *Palliat Supportive Care.* 2013;12(4):309–16.

Index

For the benefit of digital users, indexed terms that span two pages (e.g., 52–53) may, on occasion, appear on only one of those pages.

absence
  annihilation and, 40
  death/dying as an, vii–viii, 1, 28–29, 75–
    76, 131, 200–1
  my-death, other-death, and,
    xii, 20, 46
  experiences of, 131–32
  religion and, 4–5
acceptance of my-death, 206. *See also*
    neutral acceptance
Acheson, Donald, 202
Aday, Ronald, 53
addiction, 24, 82n2 *See also* smoking
adolescence, 6–8, 9–10, 15–16
adolescent sexuality, 127
after-death, xii. *See also* afterlife
  in everyday life, 138–42
  and the meaningless of life, 168, 169
afterlife, 126–32, 137–38. *See also*
    continuation/continuity: afterlife
    and; eternal life; finality of death;
    heaven; soul(s)
  vs. annihilation, 44, 128
  belief in, 42, 129, 181–82, 188, 211
    adolescents', 6–8
    as beyond thinking, 42–47
    children's, 4–5
    Christianity and, 4–5, 26–27,
      137–38, 175
    and death anxiety, 14, 43–44, 49, 54,
      124, 131, 142, 211
    and helping people embrace/engage
      with death, 82, 130
    as an "intuitive religious
      concept," 132
    my-death and, 29, 99–100, 124
    older people's, 13–14
    as proximal mechanism, 182

    religion and, 4–5, 26–27, 53, 133–34,
      138, 142n1
    religious education and, 174–75
    among terminally ill patients, 129,
      141, 152–53
    as way of avoiding or denying death,
      124, 182
  Brenda on, 8, 53, 165, 167, 168
  certainty of an, 54, 130, 170, 172
  consciousness and, 29
  as a contradiction, 99–100, 175
  empirical evidence of, 137
  everyday life and, vii
  finitude markers and, 139–41, 142,
    172, 173
  God and, 137, 167
  Heidegger on, 91
  idea of unity in, 143n15 (*see also*
    consciousness: cosmic/universal)
  as lacking boundaries, 139
  Leo on, 8, 29, 53
  Leo's rejection of the notion of, 5, 41,
    43–44, 96, 99–100, 124, 134, 136–
    37, 165, 167, 175
  Mandy on, 41–42, 126, 127, 129, 130–
    31, 132, 134, 136–37, 138, 140–41,
    165, 167, 170, 172, 188
  meaning and, 137–38, 139 (*see also*
    meaningless of life: nonexistence
    of death and the)
  Mitch Hodge on, 131
  point-of-transition and, vii, 28, 124,
    127, 132, 133, 139–40
  rhetoric and language used to discuss
    the, 137–38
  Stan on, 43–44, 165, 167, 172, 211
  transition to (*see* point-of-transition)
afterlife movement, 136

aging process, 3, 98, 107, 139. *See also* birthdays
  markers, 13, 112–13
Ahn, Eunmi, 192
ambiguities negotiated by adolescents, 6–7
Angel of Death, 48
animals, death of, xvii–xviii. *See also* pets
annihilation, 31
  vs. afterlife, 44, 128
  Brenda and, 38–39, 40, 58
  consciousness and, viii, 31, 38–39, 40–41, 164–65 (*see also* consciousness: ending of)
  continuation and, viii, 35, 40–41, 43, 44, 200–1
  fear of, 49, 58, 128, 200–1
  finality and, viii, 29–30, 38, 40, 43–44, 106
  Leo and, 38, 39, 40–41, 43, 44, 106, 128, 164–65
  my-death and, 29–30, 38–39, 40–41, 44, 48
  not even, 39–42
  nothingness and, viii, 35, 37–41, 43–44, 67, 128
  Stan and, 38–39, 40–41, 43–44, 106
  Tolstoy's struggle with the prospect of, 35
  total, 34–39, 44, 164–65, 200–1
Anthony, Sylvia, 2–3
anxiety. *See also* death anxiety; evasion; fear(s)
  continuation and, 54, 140–41, 181–82
Ardelt, Monika, 13–14
Arendt, Hannah, 119
Aries, Philippe, 7–8
art, death in, 9
Atman, 133–34
Augustine, Keith, 136, 137–38
Austin, John L., 156–57
awareness contexts, 191–92

Barad, Karen, 151
"beautiful death," 7–8
Becker, Ernest, 49, 52, 198
Being
  vs. being, 86–87
  Dasein and, 87–88, 89, 93–94
being, the structure of, 85–90

Being-unto-death, 33n13
Benore, Ethan, 129
bereavement. *See also* funeral of Aunty Sue
  and meaning, 188–89
Bering, Jesse, 131–32
Bhattacharya, Pranab, 136
Bible, 4–5
birth, 118–19
  death and, xi, 11, 96, 119, 133
birthdays, 111–12, 117
black hole, death as a, 44, 46, 82
Bluebond-Langner, Myra, 6
bodily changes, 112–13. *See also* aging process
boundaries, 91, 107, 118, 150. *See also* edgework
  bodily changes as, 112–13 (*see also* aging process)
  death and, 10, 97–98, 99, 101n15, 118, 139, 178
    death as a super-boundary/meta-boundary, 97, 99–100
  finitude and, 90, 98, 99–100, 139 (*see also* finitude)
  lack/absence of, 95, 139, 178
  Leo on, 91, 97–98, 99–100, 139
  my-death and, 82, 98, 99–100
  Stan on, 99, 118, 139
boundedness, signals that mark out our, 111. *See also* finitude marking
Brahman, 133
Brain, James, 49–50
Bregman, Lucy, 198
Bronfenbrenner, Urie, 70–71
bubble, pretense of personal immortality that forms a protective, 57
Buddhism, 133
burials, 31, 32. *See also* funeral of Aunty Sue
Butler, Judith, 157, 158, 159

Café Mortel. *See* Death Cafés
cancer
  lung, 24
  people dying from, 129, 191, 206, 208
Catlett, Joyce, 180
certainty. *See also* uncertainty
  related to death, 106

cessation, 3, 34, 36, 164–65. *See also*
consciousness: ending of;
specific topics
children, 15–16
deaths of, 21
dying, 6
growing up with death, 2–7
children's books, 4–5
Christianity, 4–5, 137
and belief in afterlife, 137–38, 175
heaven and, 4–5, 26–27, 33n12
closed awareness, 191–92
cognitive models, idealized. *See*
enabling frames
Collett, Lora-Jean, 52
communication strategies, 77–78
community involvement and
empowerment, 202–3
conditional acceptance of my-death, 206
consciousness, 34, 37, 150–51. *See also*
annihilation: consciousness and;
transposed consciousness
and continuation, 20, 34–35, 37, 40–41
cosmic/universal, 58–59, 133–34
death and, 164–65
ending of, vii, 20, 31, 34, 36, 37, 38,
40–41, 76
finitude and, 96, 109
Heidegger and, 87–88
identity and, 133–34
Leo and, 22, 26, 29, 36, 37–39, 41
my-death and, viii, 20, 29, 31, 34, 35,
76, 185
Stan on, 37–38, 40
vs. unconsciousness, 10, 34, 36
constructionism and idealism, 37
continuation/continuity, viii, 42, 106, 137–
38, 180. *See also* finality of death
absence and, viii, 20
afterlife and, 4–5, 7, 26–27, 28, 41, 44,
54, 96, 99–100, 124, 130–31, 133–
34, 136–38, 164, 167, 182 (*see also*
afterlife)
annihilation and, viii, 35, 40–41, 43,
44, 200–1
anxiety and, 54, 140–41, 181–82
Brenda on, 40, 53, 58, 75, 173
consciousness and, 20, 34–35, 37, 40–41

individual identity and, 133–34, 137–38
Leo on, 4, 28, 43, 44, 53, 75, 96, 136–37
Mandy on, 41, 125–26, 130, 136–37,
140–41, 165, 167
my-death and, xi, 20, 46, 82, 96,
99–100, 164
point-of-transition and, 124
proximal mechanisms and, 182
realism and, 37
relationships and, 58, 75, 124, 129, 130
Stan on, 43–44, 104
terminally ill children and, 6
Cozzolino, Philip, 185–86
Crettaz, Bernard, 198

Dance of Death (*danse macabre*), 9
Dasein (there-being), 87
Being and, 87–88, 89, 93–94
central function, 87–88
death and, 88–89, 102n19
Heidegger on, 87–89, 93–94, 102n19
my-death and, 88–89, 102n19
time and, 88, 89
DeArmond, Isabelle, 205
death. *See also specific topics*
of another, 20, 51–52, 75–76
attraction to, 77
learning about the nature of, 15–16
location/place of, 207–8
people's perception of how close they
are to, 13
personifications of, 48–49, 133
signals of approaching, 13 (*see also*
finitude marking)
of spouse/partner, 74–76, 129
terminology used for, 59–60, 183
death anxiety, 7, 182–84. *See also* evasion;
fear(s): of death; my-death anxiety
and belief in afterlife, 14, 43–44, 49, 54,
124, 131, 142, 211
exposure to the dying and, 204–5
death awareness movement, 198–203
Death Cafés, 198–99, 200–1, 203
"death doesn't need anything
else," 152–53
death imagery, 48–49, 127
"death is nothing to us," 197. *See also*
nothingness

death reflection, 185–86. *See also* life
        revaluation
death scales, 51–52, 53, 135–36
death studies, research, and scholarship,
        xi, 203–4, 208–11, 212–13. *See also*
        end-of-life research
defenses, symbolic, 182
denial of death, 6, 49, 52, 182, 193–94,
        198. *See also* afterlife: belief in;
        immortality; mutual pretense
Denial of Death, The (Becker), 49, 52, 198
de Quincey, Thomas, 78–79
Derrida, Jacques, 32n2, 101n15
discontinuation. *See* cessation
distal mechanisms, 182
Downey, Ann, 53
dying, xi–xii. *See also* my-dying

Eastern religion, 133
ecological systems theory. *See*
        socio-ecological theory
edgework, 9–10
education
    of end-of-life professionals,
        201–2, 207–8
    my-death, 208
    religious, 174–75
elderly. *See* old age
empathy, 15–16, 22–23, 25, 26
enabling frames, 77–82, 213, 216–17
    my-death and, 77–78, 80, 82
    nature of, 77–78, 80
    role of communication strategies in
        generating, 78
end of everything, 29–32
end-of-life, preparation for, 189–94
end-of-life care, 203–9
end-of-life research, 192, 201–2, 204–5,
        213. *See also* death studies,
        research, and scholarship
Epicurus, 197
epidemics, 1, 48
Eschleman, Andrew, 137–38
essential structures, 82, 103, 138–39.
        See also being: the structure of;
        enabling frames; finitude
    Heidegger and, 99–100, 101n7
    Leo's use of, 94, 99–100, 175

eternal life, 4–5, 27, 133, 172
euphemisms of death. *See* death:
        terminology used for
evasion, active, 54–57
existential acceptance. *See* acceptance of
        my-death
existential dilemmas, 216
existential impacts on end-of-life care
        professionals, 205
existential issues. *See also* meaning
    associated with my-death, 181–82, 186,
        205–6, 212
    communicating about, 208
    fear of death and, 186
    research on, 186, 192, 205–6, 208
    and self-awareness and growth, 186
existential psychology, 212
existential questioning, 15–16

fairy tales, 4–5
fantasies, internally generated, 136
Fear of Death Scale, 51–52
Fear of Personal Death Scale, 53
fear(s), 16, 45–46, 48, 54, 130. *See also*
        anxiety; evasion; terror
    of annihilation, 49, 58, 128, 200–1
    of death, 1–2, 45–46, 48, 50–54, 55–56,
        86, 107, 186, 190, 197, 212
        (*see also* death anxiety;
        my-death anxiety)
    cultural origins of, 49–50
    dimensions of, 33n14, 46
    Ernest Becker and, 49, 52
    forms and manifestations of,
        54, 55–56
    Mandy's, 131, 140–41, 142
    measures of (*see* death scales)
    personifications of death and, 48–49
    religious beliefs and, 52, 53–54
    uncertainty and, 197, 216
    Stan's, 45, 58, 104, 107
    of things associated with death, 54, 190
finality of death, 124. *See also* afterlife;
        continuation/continuity
    acceptance of the, 7
    annihilation and, viii, 29–30, 38, 40,
        43–44, 106 (*see also* annihilation)
    Brenda on the, 4, 5, 38, 39–40, 103

burial and, 31, 32
children's (un)awareness of the, 4, 5
Leo and, 4, 31, 32, 38, 39–40, 43–44,
    103, 128, 139, 164–65
Mandy on the, 128, 140, 165
Stan on the, 39–40, 43–44, 133, 140
finality of my-death, viii, 5, 20, 124, 140,
    164–65, 178, 181–82. *See also*
    irreversibility
finitude, 90–94
    boundaries and, 90, 98, 99–100, 139
    concept of, 90, 91, 93
    consciousness and, 96, 109
    encountered during near-death
        experiences, 107
    Heidegger on, 14, 90, 91, 92, 93–94, 98,
        102n27, 109, 110, 172
    and meaningfulness, 178, 179–80
    my-death and, 90, 92, 93, 94, 95–96,
        99–100 (*see also* finitude markers:
        my-death and)
    natal, 119
    nature of, 92
    Paul Tillich on, 98
    revisited, 105–11
finitude markers, 141
    afterlife and, 139–41, 142, 172, 173
    Brenda on, 156, 159, 173
    Leo on, 173
    Mandy and, 139–41, 142, 172, 173
    my-death and, 111, 114, 115, 116,
        119–20, 140–41, 142, 156, 159,
        172–73, 182–83
    Stan on, 120, 139, 159, 172, 173
finitude marking, 111–16
    types of, 118, 123n20
Firestone, Robert, 180
Fong, Jack, 199
Frankl, Viktor, 178
Frantz, C. M., 188–89
Freud, Sigmund, 86, 129
Freund, Alexandra, 12–13
funeral of Aunty Sue, 25–29, 30–32, 35, 85,
    170–71, 176
futurity, 19n26

Gamson and Modigliani (1989), 79–80
gender, Judith Butler on, 157, 158

general death vs. my-death, 32n2 *See also*
    my-death: vs. other-death
generative metaphors, 83n10 *See also*
    enabling frames; metaphors
Gertsman, Elina, 9
Glaser, Barney G., 191–92
God, 48, 149, 150, 152–53
    afterlife and, 137, 167
    belief in, 138, 167–68
    heaven and, 27, 152–53, 167
    Kant and, 153–54
graves, 32. *See also* funeral of Aunty Sue

hallucinations, 87, 135, 155. *See also* visions
health professionals, 201–2. *See also*
    education; hospice professionals;
    palliative care professionals
health promotion, 202–3
heart attack, Stan's, 106, 107, 120, 121, 163,
    170–71, 176, 181, 191, 218
heaven, 8, 26–27, 124, 132
    Aunty Sue and, 27–28, 30
    Brenda on, 55–56, 148–49, 152–53
    Christianity and, 4–5, 26–27, 33n12
    God and, 27, 152–53, 167
    Mandy on, 41, 128, 133, 155, 167, 175
    souls and, vii, 26–27, 53, 124, 133, 175
    Terence Nichols, 137–38
Hegel, Georg Wilhelm Friedrich, 102n30,
    154, 161n19
Heidegger, Martin, 86
    Alexandre Kojève and, 96
    on Being, 33n13, 86–88, 89, 90, 93–94
    Being and Time, 33n13, 86, 102n25
    consciousness and, 87–88
    on *Dasein*, 87–89, 93–94, 102n19
    death and, 33n13, 86, 88–89, 91, 93, 94,
        101n6, 101n15, 102n20, 110, 210
    essential structures and, 99–100, 101n7
    on existence, 87
    on finitude, 14, 90, 91, 92, 93–94, 98,
        102n27, 109, 110, 172
    Husserl and, 87
    on mortals, 89, 90
    my-death and, 90, 94, 99–100, 102n19
    Nazism and, 86
    Nothing and, 90
    time and, 87, 88

Heinämaa, Sara, 186–87
Hendrikx, David, 208–9
Hinduism, 133
Hodge, K. Mitch, 131
hospice patients. *See* terminally ill patients
hospice professionals, xvi–xvii, 201, 214–
        15n25 *See also* education; palliative
        care professionals
    personal growth associated with their
        work, 205
hospices, 201
hospitals, deaths occurring in, 207–8
Houtepen, Rob, 208–9
Husserl, Edmund, 87, 186

idealism, 37, 38–39
    constructionism and, 37
    vs. realism, 37
identity. *See also* self
    continuation/continuity and individual,
        133–34, 137–38
    relational, 67–72
immortality, 178. *See also* denial of death;
        mortality
    everyday, 58
    Kant on, 153–54
    pretense of, 57, 58–59, 60–61, 119
        (*see also* mutual pretense)
    protective bubble of everyday, 60
        bursting the, 60–64
    strategic, 57–60
    William Wordsworth and, 111
immortality belief systems, 49, 52.
        See also immortality
    Freud on, 129
immortality projects, 49
individual identity. *See* identity
individuation, 9–10
inevitability of death, 3. *See also* mortality
    Leo on the, 23–24, 77
    seen as applying to all people, 45
    Stan on the, 23–24, 25
inevitability of my-death, 48–49
    denying the, 182 (*see also* denial
        of death)
    internalization of the, 41
    Leo's encounter with the, 85
        (*see also* funeral of Aunty Sue)

intentionalism. *See* representationism
International Association for Near-Death
        Studies (IANDS), 136
interpretive packages, 79–80
irreversibility, 3, 4–5. *See also* finality
        of death

Jacques, Elliott, 12
Janoff-Bulman, R., 188–89
Jews, 48, 53
Jong, Jonathan, 53

Kant, Immanuel, 153–54
    Hegel compared with, 154
    on postulates of practical
        reason, 153–54
    representationism and, 150, 153–54
    on rhetoric, 78–79
Kellehear, Allan, 202–3
Kierkegaard, Søren, 178–79
Koestenbaum, Peter, 20
Kojève, Alexandre, 96
Korean patients in palliative
        care, 192
Kübler-Ross, Elisabeth, 198

Lee, Raymond L. M., 49–50
legacy, 168
Lester, David, 52
Levinas, Emmanuel, 67
life after death. *See* afterlife
life revaluation, 186–89
life without death, 89, 95
Lyng, Stephen, 9–10

Magid, Oren, 102n27
Mahon, Margaret, 6
Matheson, Benjamin, 137–38
McManus, Ruth, 49–50
meaning, 168–69, 186. *See also* existential
        issues; meanings
    afterlife and, 137–38, 139
    boundaries and, 95, 99, 178
        (*see also* boundaries)
    of my-death, 25, 48, 85, 96, 140, 168,
        188, 206–7, 209
    annihilation and, 38–39
    in one's life, 95, 178, 182, 183, 188–89

search for, 206 (*see also* Frankl, Viktor; meaning-making)

meaningless of life. *See also* Frankl, Viktor
after-death and the, 168, 169
bereavement and the, 188–89
fatalistic pointlessness of life and death, 8
lack of boundaries and the, 95, 139
nonexistence of death and the, 95, 106
Tolstoy on the, 35

meaning-making, 188–89, 204–5, 206

meanings, 175. *See also* meaning
of connections and relationships, 175
of death, 9, 33n14, 148, 176, 206
adolescents and, 9
impact of bereavement on, 188–89
and impacts, 173–77
instability of, 85

Melville, Herman, 60

metaphors, 78. *See also* death: terminology used for; generative metaphors

metonymy, 79–80

midlife as transition phase, 11–13

midlife crisis, 12

"mirror of nature" mentality, 151–52

missing out of expected content, 78

Moby-Dick (Melville), 60

Moraglia, Giampaolo, 179–80

mortality, xi. *See also* enabling frames; immortality; inevitability of death; my-death; *specific topics*
Anne O'Byrne on, 119
Brenda on, 118–19, 156, 166, 173
engaging with, 216
Freud on belief in, 129
intuitive knowledge of, 110
people's relationships with their, 77, 180, 206, 216
Stan on, 119, 147, 166, 171, 181

mortality salience, 182–84, 185–86

mortals, Heidegger on, 89, 90

mutual pretense, system of, 6

mutual pretense awareness, 191–92

my-death, 20. *See also* mortality; my-dying; self: death of; *specific topics*
benefits of engaging with, 178–79
life revaluation, 186–89
preparation for end-of-life, 189–94
quality of life, 179–86

conditional acceptance of, 206
as a constant companion/life companion, 62, 63, 67, 140–41, 188 (*see also* my-death relationality)
is intrinsic, 94–100
nature of, xi
vs. other-death, xi, 20, 99–100
transformation in the way Mandy engaged with, 124–26

my-death anxiety, 44, 185, 197. *See also* Becker, Ernest; death anxiety; fear(s): of death; Yalom, Irvin

my-death everywhere, 116–21

my-death relationality, 72–77, 178

my-dying, xi–xii, 127, 140–41, 179. *See also* my-death; *specific topics*

mystical experiences, 125–26, 135. *See also* spiritual encounters

mythology, 48. *See also* religion

natality and natal finitude, 119

Navigating Everyday Life: Exploring the Tension between Finitude and Transcendence (Adams), 107, 122n9

near-death experiences, 134–36, 185–86

Near-Death Experiences Scale, 135–36

negativity, 179

neutral acceptance, 189

Nichols, Terence, 137–38

Nietzsche, Friedrich, 86

Noppe, Illene, 6–7

Noppe, Lloyd, 6–7

"nothing exists beyond death," 38, 128, 168

"Nothing" (Heidegger), 90

nothingness, 37, 38. *See also* "death is nothing to us"
annihilation and, viii, 35, 37–41, 43–44, 67, 128
Brenda on, 38, 39, 158, 168
Leo on, 8, 38, 39, 44, 45, 128, 136–37, 167–68
Mandy on, 136–37, 139, 168
my-death and, xii, 35, 38–39, 46, 90, 172
negativity and, 179
Stan on, 38, 39–40, 43–44, 45, 77, 82

nurses. *See* hospice professionals; palliative care professionals

observers. *See also* transposed observer
    abiding, 25–29, 31
O'Byrne, Anne, 119
old age, 13–14, 29–30
open awareness, 191–92
other-death. *See* death: of another
"other people die," 1–2

palliative care, Korean patients in, 192
palliative care professionals, 32–33n5,
        33n6, 201, 205, 206. *See also* end-
        of-life care; hospice professionals
    Brenda's work as palliative care nurse,
        xvi–xvii, 207–8
    burnout, 204–5
    talking about their own deaths, 207–8
pandemics, 1, 48
Park, Crystal, 129
Parola, Vitor, 206
passionate suffusion, 117. *See also*
        enabling frames; finitude; my-
        death everywhere
    nature of, 82, 103
Pereira, Vera, 132
performative reality, 156–60
performative utterances, 156
pets, death of, 2–4. *See also* animals
phenomenology
    Heidegger and, 87–88
    Husserl's, 87, 186–87
phoneme regularities, 78
Plato's allegory of the cave, 149–50
point-of-transition, vii, 112–13, 126, 130,
        138–40, 175. *See also* after-death:
        in everyday life; afterlife; enabling
        frames; transition
    afterlife and, vii, 28, 124, 127, 132, 133,
        139–40 (*see also* afterlife)
    Mandy and, 124, 138–41, 175
    my-death and, 28, 58–59, 82, 124–26,
        127, 130, 131, 138–41, 163, 164
    nature of, 82, 124
    role of finitude in moments of
        transition, 122n9
    staying connected and, 132–38
posttraumatic growth, 185–86
pretense awareness, mutual, 191–92
proximal mechanisms, 182

psychoanalysis, 129
public health approach to
        dying, 202–3
public health principles, 202, 203
Pyszczynski, Tom, 182

quality of life, my-death connectivity
        and, 179–86

realism
    vs. idealism, 37
    representationism and, 147, 150
"really real" reality, 37
reason. *See under* Kant, Immanuel
reincarnation, 124, 132, 133
relational identity, 67–72
relationality, my-death, 72–77
relational processes, 151–56, 158
religion, 3, 133. *see also under* Christianity
    and belief in afterlife, 4–5, 26–27, 53,
        133–34, 138, 142n1, 174–75
    science and, 42
    and the soul, 4–5, 26–27, 133–34
religious beliefs and religiosity. *See also*
        religion
    and comfort with my-death, 52
    and fear of death, 53–54
religious experiences. *See also* mystical
        experiences; spirituality
    visions of religious figures, 135
religious language, 42, 59
    use of rhetoric in, 47n10, 84n25
representationism, 147–51, 160
    John Austin and, 156, 157
    Kant and, 150, 153–54
reuniting with loved ones, 28, 30, 128,
        129, 134
rhetoric, 78–80, 122n15
    historical perspective on, 78–79
    "new," 79
rhetorical devices, 78–80, 216
rhetorical elements in religious language,
        47n10, 84n25
Rilke, Rainer Maria, 116–17
Ring, Kenneth, 135–36
Ritter, Johannes, 12–13
Rodenbach, Rachel, 206
Rorty, Richard, 151–52

Sartre, Jean-Paul, 38–39
Saunders, Dame Cicely, 201
Scheler, Max, 110–11
Schutz, Alfred, 70
self, 186. *See also* Atman; identity
   annihilation of, 31 (*see also*
      annihilation)
   death of, 20, 51–52 (*see also* my-death)
self-esteem
   distal mechanisms and, 182
   my-death, worldviews, and, 181–83, 185
   terror management theory and, 181–83
self-generative process, 169. *See also*
      enabling frames; performative
      reality; relational processes;
      representationism
   nature of, 82, 145
self-help networks, 198, 200–1. *See also*
      Death Cafés
Sexton, James, 166–67
sexuality, 49–50, 112–13, 127
Sinclair, Shane, 180
smoking
   and death, 24–25
   and lung disease, 24–25, 182
socio-ecological theory, 70–71
soul-minus-body, 28, 53
soul(s), vii, 111, 137–38. *See also* afterlife;
      eternal life; heaven
   heaven and, vii, 26–27, 53, 124, 133, 175
   and individual identity, 133–34
   Leo, Aunt Sue, and, 27, 28, 30
   Mandy on, 41, 133, 136, 175
   my-death and, 58–59
   religion and the, 4–5, 26–27, 133–34
   Stan on, 43–44, 50–51
   Terence Nichols on, 137–38
spiritual awakenings, 135
spiritual encounters, 80. *See also* mystical
      experiences
spirituality, 138, 198, 205. *See also*
      specific topics
   and the end of life, research on, 192, 205
spouse/partner, death of, 74–76, 129
Strauss, Anselm L., 191–92
suicide, 63, 66n38, 97, 114, 127
suspected awareness, 191–92
synecdoche, 79–80

taboos around death, 49–50
terminally ill patients, 152–53. *See also*
      cancer: people dying from;
      end-of-life care
   belief in afterlife, 129, 141, 152–53
   conversations with, 145–46, 152–53
   discussing their illness, 145–46
   informing them of their terminal status,
      77, 192
   pediatric, 6
   talking to terminally ill children about
      dying, 6
   (un)awareness of their terminal
      status, 192
terror. *See also* fear(s)
   associated with my-death, 125–26, 181–
      84, 185, 186
   existential, 181–82 (*see also* existential
      issues)
terror management, 185
terror management theory, 66n31,
      181–84, 185–86
Thanatos, 48
thingafication, 151
thinking, beyond, 42–47
Tillich, Paul, 98
time
   Dasein and, 88, 89
   Heidegger and, 87, 88
time travel, 91
tobacco. *See* smoking
Tolstoy, Leo, 35
transition. *See also* midlife as transition
      phase; point-of-transition
   death as, 26, 29–30, 53, 124
   in one's relationship to my-death, xiv
transposed consciousness, 26, 29
transposed observer, 21–25, 31
trauma, 185–86
Tye, Michael, 150–51

uncertainty, 45, 88
   related to my-death, 44, 46, 124, 179,
      197, 216
unconscious beliefs regarding death, 129.
      See also Freud, Sigmund
unconsciousness vs. consciousness,
      10, 34, 36

unity. *See also* reuniting with loved ones
   in afterlife, 143n15 (*see also*
      consciousness: cosmic/universal)
universality of death, 3, 15–16

visions. *See also* hallucinations
   of religious figures, 135

Whitehead, Alfred North, 37, 154–55
Widera-Wysoczanska, Agnieszka, 188
widows. *See* spouse/partner
Wildman, Wesley J., 85

wisdom, 13–14
Woodthorpe, Kate, 210
Wordsworth, William, 111
worldviews
   distal mechanisms and, 182
   my-death, self-esteem, and, 181–83, 185
   terror management theory
      and, 181–83

Yalom, Irvin D., 86

zombies, 8–9